NEUROSCIENCE AND
SOCIAL WORK PRACTICE

*This book is dedicated to my husband, David, whose
unending support, encouragement, and love made
it possible for me to complete this book.*

NEUROSCIENCE AND SOCIAL WORK PRACTICE

The Missing Link

ROSEMARY L. FARMER

Virginia Commonwealth University

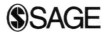

Los Angeles • London • New Delhi • Singapore • Washington DC

For information:

SAGE Publications, Inc.
2455 Teller Road
Thousand Oaks, California 91320
E-mail: order@sagepub.com

SAGE Publications India Pvt. Ltd.
B 1/I 1 Mohan Cooperative Industrial Area
Mathura Road, New Delhi 110 044
India

SAGE Publications Ltd.
1 Oliver's Yard
55 City Road
London EC1Y 1SP
United Kingdom

SAGE Publications Asia-Pacific Pte. Ltd.
33 Pekin Street #02-01
Far East Square
Singapore 048763

Library of Congress Cataloging-in-Publication Data

Farmer, Rosemary L.
Neuroscience and social work practice : the missing link / Rosemary L. Farmer.
    p. cm.
Includes bibliographical references and index.
ISBN 978-1-4129-2697-3 (cloth)
ISBN 978-1-4129-2698-0 (pbk.)
    1. Medical social work. 2. Neurosciences. 3. Social service. I. Title.

HV687.F37 2009
362.1′0425—dc22

                                                    2008026112

08   09   10   11   12   10 9 8 7 6 5 4 3 2 1

Acquisitions Editor:	Kassie Graves
Editorial Assistant:	Veronica Novak
Production Editor:	Catherine M. Chilton
Copy Editor:	Youn-Joo Park
Typesetter:	C&M Digitals (P) Ltd.
Proofreader:	Doris Hus
Indexer:	Diggs Publishing Services
Cover Designer:	Edgar Abarca
Marketing Manager:	Carmel Schrire

Contents

Acknowledgments

A lthough a book may have one author, many people help to make it a reality. I wish to mention these people:

Sage editor Kassie Graves, whose interest and encouragement provided ongoing sustenance.

Former Sage editor Art Pomponio, who made it possible for me to begin the book journey.

Professor Edward Taylor, my neuroscience mentor since my doctoral student days when I spent two semesters studying with him at the National Institutes of Health Neuropsychiatric Research Center at St. Elizabeth's Hospital in Washington, DC.

My clients, who consistently provide the impetus for thinking about new ways of helping persons manage their chronic illnesses.

My social work graduate students, who listened enthusiastically to the neuroscience content I was learning and writing about.

1

Linking to the Neuroscientific Revolution

Neuroscience is a missing link for social work. Neuroscience is the science of the brain or the science(s) of the nervous system(s). It is a missing link for human service specialists such as social workers, psychotherapists, psychologists, psychiatric nurses, educators, child care workers, and others who work with people. It is argued in this chapter that there are at least six reasons why human service professionals should embrace the missing link.

These six reasons (to which we'll return later) are as follows:

1. A neuroscientific revolution has occurred. Although this revolution may not provide all the answers, it needs to be acknowledged and understood.

2. Neuroscientific insights can be of immediate and direct benefit in improving our understanding of human behavior and practice.

3. The probability is that neuroscience over time will yield additional powerful insights, and we must be ready—intellectually, emotionally, and institutionally—to understand these developments.

4. Neuroscience is enhancing our understanding of what it is to be human; the relevance of this will depend on whether one's conception of social work is narrow or broad.

5. Neuroscience can help social workers and other human service professionals to cope with the increasing professional difficulties they face; clinical practice is becoming more difficult, as practitioners encounter an increasing complexity of human and societal problems and diagnoses.

6. Human service professionals should aspire to contribute to neuroscientific understanding by engaging more fully in cross-disciplinary study and by developing more comprehensive conceptualizations—the hallmark of social work intervention—of psychosocial adaptation.

A missing link is something, hitherto unknown, that is necessary to solve a problem, to complete a series. The link is often described as a missing item of knowledge that, when recognized and understood, explains how living entities have evolved from others. It can apply to all kinds of living entities such as flowering plants; it is more traditionally used in referring to hominid evolution. Just as the understanding of humans is incomplete without any such missing link or links, the understanding of human thinking, emotion, and behavior is similarly incomplete without including the insights from neuroscience. While biology alone is not destiny, the biological (i.e., the brain) dimension is crucial. While neuroscience does not provide the whole picture, and much remains to be discovered, it provides an important missing piece to our knowledge and understanding.

This book specifies a framework for human service professionals to understand, and to contribute to, the neurosciences. It also explains and illustrates the specifics of how the missing link can enhance specific therapeutic situations. Knowledge of brain sciences is necessary for human service professionals such as social workers, and this missing link will transform existing thinking and practices in important respects. As an example, our ability to work more effectively with those who have endured trauma is enhanced by new knowledge about the different types of memory and where they are located in the brain. Our understanding of autism has been enlarged by the very recent discovery of mirror neurons, which help to explain how an infant learns to be in relationships with others—a skill that appears deficient in persons with autism.

As an introduction, this chapter sketches the nature of neuroscience, suggests why human service disciplines should embrace the missing link, outlines social neuroscience, discusses four levels of social work interaction with social neuroscience, and indicates the contents of the remaining chapters. The levels of interaction with social neuroscience (each being discussed later) are as follows:

- advocating,
- fundamental understandings,
- policy-relevant understandings, and
- client practice-level understandings.

Linking

Why should social workers and other human service professionals embrace the missing link of neuroscience? Reconsider the six reasons just given.

Reason 1

The first reason is that the world is not as it was. There has been a neuro-scientific revolution. Fundamental discoveries are clarifying the role of the brain in helping to shape and condition behavior, thought, and emotion (see Figure 1.1). We now have better understanding and opportunities for action about human functioning across the broadest range! The Decade of the Brain (1990-1999) and the Human Genome Project (1990-2003)—and other developments such as talk of the coming "neurosociety"—symbolize the importance of this neuroscientific revolution.

The Decade of the Brain had the aim, as noted in the presidential proclamation inaugurating the project, of enhancing "public awareness of the benefits to be derived from brain research" (Project on the Decade of the Brain, 2000). Authorizing the Decade of the Brain, the U.S. Senate Joint Resolution (1990) noted the scale of neuroscience's relevance, the relevance of neuroscience for particular disorders, and the potential for understanding human behavior and feelings in general. It also pointed to the fact that 15 of

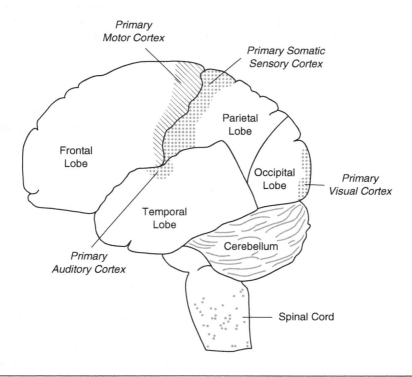

Figure 1.1   The Brain

the Nobel prizes in medicine or physiology over the past quarter century had been awarded to neuroscientists.

On a scale of relevance, the Congressional Resolution claimed that approximately 50 million Americans are affected by disorders and disabilities that involve the brain; that the treatment costs are $305 billion annually; and that the incidence of neurological, psychiatric, psychological, and cognitive disorders among older persons will increase as the number of older persons increases. On the relevance of neuroscience to particular disorders, the Congressional resolution picked out the significance of neuroscientific research for some forms of mental retardation; for inheritable neurological disorders like Huntington's disease and mental disorders like affective illnesses (with the hope that mapping biochemical circuitry will permit the rational design of potent medications, with minimal side effects); for Parkinson's, schizophrenia, and Alzheimer's disease. This is a shortened list; for instance, the Congressional resolution (U.S. Senate Joint Resolution, 1990) added another "whereas" clause to the effect that

> studies of the brain and central nervous system will contribute not only to the relief of neurological, psychiatric, psychological, and cognitive disorders, but also to the management of fertility and infertility, cardiovascular disease, infectious and parasitic diseases, developmental disabilities and immunological disorders, as well as to an understanding of behavioral factors that underlie the leading, preventable causes of death. (p. 2)

That was written in the 1990s, and the growth of research achievements since then has accelerated.

The Human Genome Project set out to identify all the genes in human DNA and to determine the sequences of the some 3 billion pairs of bases that constitute this DNA (see Figure 1.2). Like the Decade of the Brain, this project was administered by the U.S. government.

The Human Genome Project was completed in 2003. The scientific aims of the Human Genome Project were achieved 2 years before the scheduled deadline, including the unexpected finding that the human genome has only about 30,000 genes and not the 100,000 originally predicted. (It is also important to note that one third of the 30,000 human genes are expressed in the brain.) The project succeeded in identifying all the human DNA and in determining the sequences of pairs of bases that make up this DNA. A genome is the totality of an organism's DNA, and that includes the genes, which provide instructions that dictate the making of particular proteins. The proteins are important because they are said to determine the functioning and behavior of the organism. The genetic instructions are written in a four-letter code, which refers to bases or chemicals that are abbreviated as A, T, C, and G. The ordering of these bases is significant because it determines even whether the organism is human, which is of significant consequence. The Human Genome Project also had

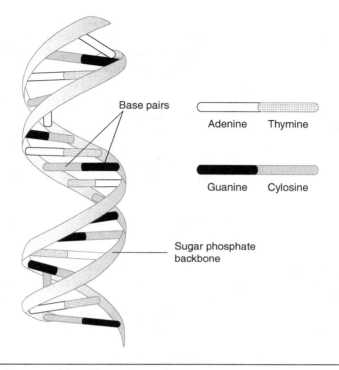

Base pairs

Adenine   Thymine

Guanine   Cylosine

Sugar phosphate
backbone

Figure 1.2   Double Helix

other objectives. One (which some might find regrettable) was transferring these technologies to the private sector, where financial gain may be more important than human benefit. Another was to address the ethical, legal, and social issues of the Project—called, in bureaucratese, the ELSI issues (also known as ethical, legal, and social issues).

Benefits from the results of the Human Genome Project in terms of molecular medicine have clear relevance for why social work should embrace the missing link. Claims have been made for improvements in molecular medicine in terms of better disease diagnosis; identification of genetic predispositions to particular diseases; gene therapy; and control systems for drugs, pharmacogenomic "custom drugs," and the rational drug design mentioned above (Oak Ridge National Laboratory, n.d.). Yet other benefits had less or no claim on social work attention (e.g., benefits for bioarchaeology and livestock breeding).

The coming neurosociety is another development symbolic of the neuroscience revolution. Restak (2006) is among those who forecast the arrival of a neurosociety, an example of other developments symbolizing the revolution: "During the first half of the twenty-first century our understanding of the human brain will revolutionize how we think about ourselves and our interactions with other people. . . . What's more, our evolving knowledge about the brain has led to the new discipline of social neuroscience: the application of brain science to social interactions. This represents a dramatic break from our usual ways of looking at human behavior" (pp. 1-3). For social workers, who have always been keenly interested in human behavior, and for whom the *social* is paramount, this "brave new world" that Restak describes must be heeded. Social relationships and social support are often integral to the interventions social workers provide, and appreciating where in the brain (and how) the social takes place (e.g., how the right brain of the parent links up with the right brain of the infant) can enhance our ability to aid persons in their social interactions.

The Five Further Reasons for Embracing the Missing Link

Reason 2

The second reason for embracing the missing link, as noted earlier, is that neuroscientific insights can be of immediate and direct benefit in improving our understanding of human behavior and practice. Supplementing the examples from the Decade of the Brain and the Human Genome Project, the following chapters offer specific examples of the recent neuroscience research that affects our practice (e.g., the research that has used magnetic resonance imaging [MRI] to scan the living brain and provide answers to some of the mysteries of human behavior; and neurobiological findings related to work with children, adolescents, and their families, especially in the child welfare and school settings). The applications discussed are of both micro and macro relevance. Despite the adjectives *immediate* and *direct*, social work professional skill and ingenuity is needed in applying the insights in varying and specific situations.

Let's consider an example of what is immediately relevant. As we develop psychosocial assessments and plan interventions, we are always interested in the person's past and present behavior, some of which is usually causing the problems that result in the person seeing a social worker or another human service professional. Although we have routinely looked at the psychological and the social aspects of behavior, we have paid scant attention to the biological aspects. The neurosciences provide some of the missing biological data that we need to perform fuller and more meaningful bio-psycho-social-spiritual assessments. Instead of merely listing gender, race, age, and so forth in the biological section, we can now add biological risk factors such as trauma and attachment difficulties. As we increase our understandings of problems that adversely affect the brain and nervous system, we are better prepared to provide remedies and/or management strategies for chronic and unremitting problems.

Reason 3

Reason 3—that neuroscience over time will yield additional insights—suggests that social workers should prepare themselves for this. Chapter 3 offers the transactional model, which focuses on the biological/psychological/social/ spiritual domains of human behavior. It is suggested that this model will aid in our intellectual and emotional preparation for the insights to come. Beyond this, there is the matter of institutional openness and to changed ways of thinking and knowing. For example, in several of my published works and professional presentations, I have attempted to present basic psychopharmacology knowledge for all human service professionals, not just those who work in the area of mental health. This content has been well received, though usually questioned as to why those who work in school and social service settings need to know this information. The world of practice is not as neatly dichotomized as it was in the past, so that school social workers and child welfare workers (as well as social workers in mental health) need to know about psychotropic medications and findings that add to our knowledge about which medications work for whom. They need to be alert to future findings, because inevitably there will be even more helpful data to share.

Reason 4

The fourth reason for embracing the Missing Link is that neuroscience has contributed—and will continue to contribute—to a better understanding of what it is to be human. Social workers have always been interested in human behavior, and in fact, all professionally educated social workers take at least several human behavior and social environment courses. Yet, what appears relevant in this respect depends on whether one's conception of social work is narrow or broad. Members of practice-oriented disciplines such as social work, counseling, and nursing typically face the dilemma of how to broaden their perspective beyond what has traditionally seemed to work, beyond the little fiefdoms that make up traditional social work and the other traditional subdivisions of the human service spectrum. For a discipline such as social work, which is grounded in human behavior, such insights as are available from neuroscience on the intricacies of brain function are significant. More than neuroscientific insights and data are needed for some issues, of course. For instance, there's the matter of mind, which needs the input not only of Neuroscience but also of Philosophy of Mind. With that proviso, it is helpful to learn more about the brain and the mind through neuroscience and analyze how these two constructs are related and interact. Is the mind an expression of the functioning of the brain, as some believe (Kandel, 1979), or can the mind be seen as being "at the interface of interpersonal experience and the structure and function of the brain," as Siegel (1999, p. 3) proposes? For example, what does it mean when someone says "she is out of her mind" or "he is not in his right mind?"

Reason 5

The fifth reason for embracing the missing link is that neuroscience can help social workers and other human service professionals manage the increasing difficulties that they face as practitioners. The job is becoming more complicated, as practitioners encounter the challenges of multiple problems and diagnoses and work in an increasingly complex and stressful world. Often, we feel less than confident in our ability to help ameliorate these problems. Whereas the social worker of three decades ago might encounter a client with 1 diagnosis and 10 problems, now it is just as likely to have a client with 5 diagnoses and 30 problems. One of my own clients, for instance, suffers from Attention Deficit Hyperactivity Disorder (ADHD), depression, anorexia, bipolar disorder, and personality disorder. Knowing about the brain and its influence on all bodily functions, as well as the psychological, social, and spiritual aspects of a person, helps to provide a fuller conceptualization of the challenges being faced by this person and how to recognize and use all of the person's strengths. It is true that overdiagnosing may now be more prevalent, but it is unlikely to account for the totality of the increase nowadays in complexity. This increasing complexity is also recognized in the literature (e.g., Farmer, Bentley, & Walsh, 2006). Neuroscience can help us to understand the etiology of such complexity and therefore how better to intervene.

Reason 6

The sixth reason is that social workers should aspire to contribute to neuroscientific understanding; we are equipped to do this. The example given above was to engage more fully in cross-disciplinary study and to develop more comprehensive understanding of psycho-social adaptation. This will seem strange to some social workers, as neuroscience is conceptualized as hard science. Despite social work's century-long quest to be considered as a scientifically based discipline and the inclusion of quantitative approaches (as well as qualitative), most social workers enter their profession because they are less than totally enamored of "hard science" and more interested in the human sciences. The transactional model, just mentioned and as discussed in chapter 3, suggests an approach for holistic social work contributions. Supplementing that, perhaps we can learn from those in psychology (and in social science disciplines) who have expressed research interest in social neuroscience. Daniel Siegel, a child psychiatrist who is considered to be an expert on the neurobiology of childhood attachment, and whose writings and presentations bridge the gap between neuroscience research and clinical practice, refers to the social nature of the brain. For Siegel (1999), this means that social relationships (via attachment) are necessary for the development of the brain, and social experiences of the developing child determine how neurons connect to each other. Social workers and other human service professionals, who frequently deal with the social dimension of their clients' lives, have not traditionally considered the social as having anything to do with the brain. Others are talking about social neuroscience, and we should turn toward it also.

   Is the embrace of the missing link optional for social work professionals who want to achieve effective results? I think not. I'm saying this because I would not want these six reasons for linking to be seen as mere advantages that can be taken or left. The neuroscientific revolution, properly interpreted, is real and here to stay, and we need to be engaged in it.

What's Neuroscience, in a Nutshell?

Today, the neurosciences comprise a broad array of disciplines that are focused on understanding the brain and the nervous system, and they are critical links in advancing understanding of human thought, emotion, and behavior. In other words, neuroscience is an interdisciplinary undertaking that operates at several levels (i.e., the molecular, the cellular, the systemic, the behavioral, and the cognitive). The molecular level is the most elementary and includes the many different molecules that make up brain matter and "play many different roles that are crucial for brain function" (Bear, Connors, & Paradiso, 2007, p. 13). The cellular level concerns neurons; the different types of neurons, their functions, and how they become "wired together." The systemic level is about distinct brain circuits that are formed from groups of neurons and perform a specific function (e.g., visual or motor). The behavioral level describes how specific neural systems work in concert to produce integrated behaviors. The most complex level of analysis, the cognitive, is concerned with neural mechanisms that mediate higher forms of mental activity, such as self-awareness and language. Although the term is defined in different ways (e.g., study of the brain, study of the nervous system, the latter including not only the central nervous system of brain and spinal cord but also the peripheral nervous system), neuroscience includes study of how the brain and nervous system(s) mediate thinking, behavior, and feelings.

   Neuroscience encompasses a large variety of specialties. Experimental neuroscientists, for example, include developmental neurobiologists (they analyze the development and maturation of the brain), molecular neurobiologists (they use the genetic material of neurons to understand structure and function of brain molecules), computational neuroscientists (who use mathematics and computers to develop models of brain functions), neuroanatomists (who study the structure of the nervous system), neuroethologists (they study the neural basis of specific animal behaviors), neurochemists (they study the chemistry of the nervous system), neurophysiologists (they measure the electrical activity in the nervous system), neuropharmacologists (who examine the effects of drugs on the nervous system), psychophysicists (who measure perceptual abilities quantitatively), and physiological psychologists (who study the biological basis of behavior). Others include clinical specialists such as neuropathologists (they find changes in nervous system tissue that result from disease), neurosurgeons (perform surgery on the brain and spinal cord), psychiatrists (physicians who diagnose and treat mental disorders), and neurologists (physicians who diagnose and treat diseases of the nervous system).

Choice of a beginning date for neuroscience can be disputed, as for many other subjects. Some might want to choose an event in ancient history, perhaps tipping one's hat to Herodotus and Galen. A more promising choice is the 17th century, following the contribution of Rene Descartes—physiologist as well as philosopher and mathematician. Important advances were made in subsequent years. In the 19th century, for instance, Paul Broca and others provided evidence of the localization of functions in different parts of the brain; and Charles Darwin spoke to the evolution of nervous systems. In 1906, as another example, Camillo Golgi and Santiago Ramon y Cajal won the Nobel Prize for medicine and physiology: Golgi's staining technique led to a reconceptualization of the brain as composed of different cellular elements. The Golgi technique is still used today.

The term *neuroscience* itself came into use in the late 1950s and became more widely accepted in the early 1960s as the Neurosciences Research Program was developed at the Massachusetts Institute of Technology. In 1969, as the Society for Neuroscience was founded, the field became firmly established within the academic discipline of Life Sciences. Attendance at the Society for Neuroscience's annual conference now exceeds 30,000, a large increase over the 1,396 attendees in 1971.

Social Neuroscience

It is recommended that social workers particularly focus on social neuroscience. This involvement would not, of course, preclude engagement in the activity of other "basic science" levels of neuroscience. Although social neuroscience is currently ensconced mainly within the field of psychology (the 2005 Conference of the American Psychological Society featured a keynote address on the social brain), social work also can benefit from engaging social neuroscience. After all, to date we have made extensive use of concepts and theories from psychology to enhance our psychosocial perspective, so in some ways, this will be a natural extension of our theoretical frame of reference.

What is social neuroscience? At what levels of understanding should the interaction between social work and social neuroscience take place? (i.e., what levels of linkage?)

What Is Social Neuroscience?

The term *social neuroscience* was introduced in 1992 to describe a field of research—or set of fields—using social and biological levels of analysis (Cacioppo & Berntson, 1992). It is an emerging field that studies links between social processes and neurosciences. It analyzes concepts and ideas from the neural to the social level (Ito & Cacioppo, 2001). Because there is such an assortment of study areas, I use the term *social neuroscience* here in a symbolic sense to refer to a variety of disciplinary titles, including cognitive neuroscience, affective neuroscience, neuropsychology, and neuropsychiatry—as well as social neuroscience. The assortment goes on, each specialty with its own journals and literature. Generally, social neuroscience is concerned with the neurological features associated with the processes that have traditionally been studied in social psychology, and it is closely related to cognitive neuroscience and affective neuroscience.

Social workers and other human service professionals, who frequently deal with the social dimension of their clients' lives, have not traditionally considered the social as having anything to do with the brain. As psychosocial practitioners, we have been remiss in that we have not fully appreciated the significance of the bio-social aspects of development. Our nonmedical background makes it unlikely that we will ever be specialists in the area of neuroscience, but social aspects of human behavior have always been a large part of the social work approach to human problems.

The current objective of social neuroscience is to understand the relationship between the brain and social interaction. *Social neuroscience* has been defined as "the exploration of the neurological underpinnings of the processes traditionally examined by, but not limited to, social psychology" (Decety & Keenan, 2006). In their introduction to the first issue of their new journal specifically intended to disseminate research and ideas on social neuroscience, editor Decety and deputy editor Keenan explained that

> [in] the past decade a new and exciting academic domain has expanded to scientifically explore the biological mechanisms of social interaction. This rapid growth is reflected in various ways, including new graduate programs, handbooks . . . textbooks . . . as well as special issues of different journals.

Decety and Keenan (2006) went on to declare that, "with roots in many disciplines, including but not limited to neuroscience, social psychology, developmental science, economics, and cognitive psychology, social neuroscience has come of age" (p. 1). It is interesting to note that social neuroscience as an academic domain has expanded to include the biological aspects of social interaction only during the past 10 years.

It is perhaps unfortunate—and I agree—that descriptions of social neuroscience should speak in terms of "underpinnings." That gives the unnecessary impression that the biological component is the more fundamental. Yet it is natural, if regrettable, overenthusiasm, especially when neurobiological find-ings are providing catalytic changes in existing disciplines. The academic activity in the "new" field is impressive. Using stock market terminology, it is a growth discipline.

Decety and Keenan (2006) are referring to what I call an "assortment of dis-ciplines." Social work is implicated in some of these, and we might consider the impact on the disciplines close to social work. Take the clinical example. Social workers have always looked toward the medical profession, and during the 20th century, we closely identified with physicians and psychiatrists, and alternatively have attempted to disassociate ourselves from the tenets of the medical model. During the 1920s and 1930s, psychiatry in the United States became increasingly influenced by psychoanalysis, and many social workers who worked with psychiatrists were also influenced by the emerging field of psychoanalysis. More recently, psychoanalysts are being influenced by research findings from the neurosciences. There is a bridging of the former divide between biological psychiatry (somatic treatments) and psychoanalytic practitioners (the psychological). The term *neuropsychoanalysis* is now being used to describe the integration of mind and brain and to appreciate the possible connection between some of Freud's ideas and those of modern neuroscience (Altman, 2003; Solms, 2000; Wolfe, 2003).

In speaking of social neuroscience, I am using the term in a generic sense rather than a bureaucratic sense of endorsing a particular institution. I do not intend to exclude variations and overlappings that sometimes go by different names. For instance, some have spoken of social cognitive neuroscience, which seeks to understand human behaviors and attitudes by involving neuroscien-tists with social psychologists, cognitive psychologists, anthropologists, neurol-ogists, sociologists, and others. Social cognitive neuroscience has also been described as—repeating the metaphor—"a really hot growth area" (see Azar, 2002; Ochsner & Lieberman, 2001).

Levels of Linkage

At what levels should we interact? I discuss here four levels of interaction between social work and social neuroscience, those listed earlier in this chapter. Significant social work benefits accrue from social neuroscience in terms of the following levels:

Level 1: advocating neuroscientific research issues of greatest relevance to social work clients

Level 2: participating in identifying fundamental understandings

Level 3: developing neuroscientifically informed understandings relevant to making recommendations on policy making

Level 4: deepening understandings, also neuroscientifically informed, that will help in coping with the serious problems that clients bring

The four levels are not offered as separate and distinct; they interweave and the categories are deconstructible. For example, the most general of the levels also relates to, and overlaps with, the least general. Also, the examples operate at several of the levels. The intention in describing the four levels is merely to indicate the range of possibilities for interactions between social work and social neuroscience.

Social workers approaching social neuroscience can apply their own methods at each of these levels, such as case studies. Decety and Keenan (2006) point to the value of human case studies, for example, observing the relationship between social behavior and neurological systems. The case study has long been an important tool used in social work. Recall that Sigmund Freud relied heavily on human case studies, and he (who wanted to be a biologically based physician) has been a model for social workers for the past century. Freud developed conclusions in his case studies not only for the particular patient but also—in his profound theorizing—for human behavior in general.

An example of how different levels of analysis are integrated in the field of social neuroscience can be seen in the study of drug abuse and addiction. Using the biological level of analysis as defined earlier, data about the opiate system in the brain are studied, and this includes information about how drugs lead to opiate receptor changes, which ultimately contribute to drug tolerance and addiction. From the social level of analysis, researchers look at the social context of the individual who is using the drug (i.e., economics, opportunity, peer-group influences, and family dynamics). By looking at this problem through a lens of multiple determinism, a much richer analysis and eventual understanding ensues.

Level 1: Advocating neuroscience research questions. Some scientific research questions are of greater relevance than other questions to social work clients, and social workers should accept this traditional advocacy role—for the benefit of our clients—in relation to the neuroscientific revolution. Examples are suggested in the following chapters and include the areas of trauma, psychotherapy, and psychotropic medications. As an example, how can new knowledge about the developing brain during childhood help us to find more effective psychosocial interventions for children with ADHD and other biobehavioral disorders?

Other neuro–social-science disciplines accept this advocacy role for themselves. Both those involved in neuroeconomics and neuro–political-science, for example, attempt a two-way relationship with neuroscience. The 2006 Fourth Annual Conference of the Neuroeconomics Society set up its agenda on this two-directional basis. Neuroeconomics seeks understandings from neuroscience; it also aims to offer neuroscience sounder mathematical understandings. Glimcher (2003) describes neuroscience as failing to adequately incorporate probability theory in his book subtitled *The Science of Neuroeconomics:* "Mathematical theories of decision making that include probability theory must form the core of future approaches to understanding the relationship between behavior and brain, because understanding the relationship between behavior and brain is fundamentally about understanding decision making" (pp. 177-178). From neuroscience, neuro–political-scientists seek information on topics such as decision making, motivation, emotion, and stereotyping. In the other direction, some neuro–political-scientists want to shape the choice of research questions (e.g., focusing on the political). For example, the 2006 Annual Meeting of the American Society of Political Science contained a panel on "neuroscientific advances in the study of political science" (Alford, 2006), including significant topics such as the neurological basis of representative democracy (Hibbing & Alford, 2006), neuroscience and analytical narratives (Schiemann, 2006), and considerations on the neuroscience of power (Valk & Parisi, 2006). A few neuro–political-scientists even work directly with functional magnetic resonance imaging (imaging the workings of the living brain); they aren't limited to passive using. I mention this only because it is suggestive of the range of the interest (Alford, 2006) in using neuroscience understandings and methodologies among disciplines that have not traditionally been allied with the neurosciences.

Level 2: Fundamental understandings. At this most general level, social workers can benefit from participating in identifying fundamental insights about human behavior, thinking, and emotions. As one example, there is the question of the meaning—the implications—of a neuroscientific view that we are emotional beings who think, rather than thinking beings who have emotions (e.g., see LeDoux, 1996). Barring brain injury or malformation, a human nonemotional moment is a fiction. As Restak (2006) puts it, "Neuroscience is suggesting here that we must change our ideas about reason, rationality, and what it means to be emotional. . . . Thinking and emotionality are inextricably intertwined" (pp. 51-52). We might also consider the neuroscientific views about the brain's sensory systems being "narcissistic" (e.g., see Atkins, 1996), and about the brain being wired to lie in, for instance, the anterior cingulate gyrus (e.g., see Tancredi, 2005, pp. 119-121). What does this mean for purely rational, purely objective judgments? Social workers have access to large numbers of clients, often over long periods of time, and this puts us in an ideal position to study thinking and emotions, and their interconnections, among various persons. Other examples might include the relation of genes to behavior and the realignment of conceptual frameworks in terms of neural signatures.

Social neuroscience includes tracking the neural signatures of human behavior, thoughts, and feelings. This tracking concerns, for instance, "sophisticated mental states such as truth versus lie, veridical versus false memory, style of moral reasoning or the likelihood of aggressive behavior" (Decety & Keenan, 2006, p. 6). In schizophrenia research, neural tracking has been used extensively (via MRI and function MRI [fMRI] brain scans) to decipher the structural and functional brain abnormalities that exist in this illness. With regard to schizophrenia, enlarged ventricles (fluid-filled cavities in the brain) and cortical atrophy (signifying loss of neurons) are found in the brains of some persons with schizophrenia and can be considered neural correlates of this illness. Farmer and Pandurangi (1997) used magnetic resonance imaging and CT scans to compare two groups of persons with schizophrenia, those with and those without brain impairment. Their study adds support for the deconstruction of the concept of schizophrenia, suggesting that it is not best understood as a unitary concept—the way that the concept has been constructed. Rather, schizophrenia is described as a heterogeneous illness. In other words, not everyone with schizophrenia looks or acts the same, and the brains of persons with schizophrenia do not look the same on scans (structural or functional anomalies may or may not be seen). In recent years, researchers have investigated the neural correlates (i.e., neural signatures) of bilingualism, self-consciousness, and autobiographical memory. Another example is a study by Krendl, Macrae, Kelley, Fugelsang, and Heatherton (2006) that investigated the functional anatomic correlates (e.g., amygdala, insula, anterior cingulate, and lateral prefrontal cortex) related to how judgments are formed about those who have characteristics known to be stigmatizing (e.g., obesity, facial piercing, transsexuality, and unattractiveness). This study provides a beginning understanding of the neural underpinnings of stigma. Another study (Haas, Omura, Amin, Constable, & Canli, 2006) examined the temporal dynamics of networks of structures associated with particular personality traits. Still other studies concern the visual analysis of human actions (Chouchourelou, Matsuka, Harber, & Shiffrar, 2006) and self-related processing in the sexual domain (Heinzel et al., 2006). Relevant concerns are also reflected in "the basic premise behind" social cognitive neuroscience. Azar (2002) describes this premise as infusing "social psychology with brain science methodology in the hopes of deciphering how the brain controls such cognitive processes as memory and attention, which then influence social behaviors such as stereotyping, emotions, attitudes and self-control."

Social workers should be equipped to collaborate appropriately with others who are also concerned with such fundamental understandings. For example, neurophilosophy applies neuroscienctific concepts to traditional philosophical questions. An example of an exciting neurophilosophical issue is the nature of a unified self. Social workers have been involved with self psychology since the 1970s, when Heinz Kohut began to formulate this new theory about what is required for the development of a cohesive self. Several social work clinicians in the Chicago area have been closely involved with the ongoing development of this theory (Elson, 1986; Palombo, 1985). Other examples include the nature of psychological states (e.g., emotions, beliefs, and desires) and of perceptual knowledge. Neurophilosophy is usually distinguished from philosophy of neuroscience. The latter is concerned with foundational issues in neuroscience (e.g., descriptive, normative, and constructive questions about the nature of neuroscientific explanations). The exchange between neuroscience and philosophy, in an ideal world, thus would be bidirectional—the same ideal as intended in the neuropolitical and neuroeconomic (e.g., see Churchland, 1986, 2002).

Level 3: Policy-relevant understandings. The more familiar—and less general—level of understanding would include using thoughtful neuroscientific results as part of "considered policy making around controversial issues" (Decety & Keenan, 2006, p. 6), offering "new perspectives and tools for policymakers willing to use them." Decety and Keenan use addiction as their example, and that is a topic discussed in chapter 7, where we consider addiction as a brain-based mental illness. In this vein, it could be argued that more resources are needed for treatment of persons who become biologically addicted to a substance than for the building and maintenance of prisons. For other examples, there is the mass of social and political issues that result from completion of the Human Genome Project, noted above.

Social workers should be well placed to understand policy-relevant issues in the post–genomic age—the period after completion of the Human Genome Project. The ELSI program within the Human Genome Project identified some nine areas that raise social concerns (U.S. Department of Energy, n.d.); I include only some as examples of policy-relevant areas as follows:

- Fairness, privacy, and confidentiality in the use of genetic information are concerns, and this includes concerns about genetic discrimination in insurance coverage and in the workplace. Social workers should be able to advise and advocate for clients on questions such as who should have access to personal genetic information and who owns and controls genetic information; for instance, how should such information be used, if at all, by the courts, schools, and adoption agencies?
- Psychological impact and stigmatization is another set of questions raised by the ELSI program. Social workers are in a good position to be able to advise on how genetic information affects society's perceptions of an individual, how genetic information affects individuals who are members of minority communities, and how to assist clients in managing stigma when it does occur.
- Another issue is the use of genetic information in reproductive decisions and reproductive rights (e.g., about the risks and limitations of genetic technology).
- The uncertainties associated with gene tests constitute another area. For example, there is the issue of whether genetic testing should be performed when no treatment is available and whether minor children should be tested for adult-onset diseases. Again, these are all issues that social workers need to be prepared to help their clients address.

Level 4: Client practice-level understandings. More specific would be the benefits of neuroscientific findings for purposes such as working with clients with dysfunctional human bonding or relationship issues associated with, for example, impulsivity in decision making (or judgment). Examples include decision making involving antisocial behaviors, couple relationships, and certain medical afflictions. Social workers have historically worked with persons who experience environmental deprivations as well as serious emotional and psychiatric problems, and social neuroscience is a resource for such work. The relevance and scope here is suggested in a discussion by Fisher, Aron, and Mashek (2002) concerning three primary emotion-motivation systems that have evolved in the brains of mammals and birds for mating, reproduction, and parenting. It argues that each system is associated with neural correlates and behavior repertoire. The study claims that the evolution of these emotion-motivation systems "contribute to contemporary patterns of marriage, adultery, divorce, remarriage, stalking, homicide and other crimes of passion, and clinical depression due to romantic rejection" (Fisher et al., 2002, p. 416). Neuroscientific explanations are also relevant for social workers concerned with the criminal justice system. Antisocial behavior and day-to-day impulsivity attitudes are frequently studied in connection with criminal behavior, and knowledge gained from these studies would be useful to those who work with criminal offenders.

There is a neurobiological component in impulsivity and antisociality, to be sure. As an example of the relevance of neuroscientific factors, prefrontal lobe abnormalities are among other biological factors implicated (Bechara & Bar-On, 2006). Studies have shown that low levels of serotonin are associated with impulsive and aggressive behaviors, also perhaps associated with depression. Persons who have low levels of serotonin are impulsive in the sense that they have little regard for the longer term consequences of their actions. They are aggressive in that there might be violence against others or, in the form of suicide, against the person himself or herself. The mechanism of serotonin is not completely understood currently, as the reader might expect.

There is a strong genetic component to antisocial behavior. Although warning against "genetic etiology," Lisa Cohen (2005) points to this component and reports that estimates of the genetic contribution range from a low of about a third (compared with other "environmental" components) to a high of almost 70%. Among the many issues that Cohen discusses is that "animal research and studies of healthy humans also point to potential lines of investigation, specifically into the relationship between oxytocin, vasopressin and the reward circuitry as well as the integration of cortico-limbic circuitry in antisocial individuals" (p. 118).

Also at this more specific level, neuroscientific findings have relevance for social work and all clinical practice with a large number of persons with specific illnesses. These understandings can be used for all kinds of interventions. Consider some kinds of mental retardation and recall the role that impoverished environments play in some cases. There can be a failure of normal circuits to form in the brain as associated with mental retardation. It has also been established that normal synaptic development, including dendritic spines, depends on a rich early environment. Examples of other particular illnesses include eating disorders, depression, posttraumatic stress disorder (PTSD),

Alzheimer's, phobia, Tourette's syndrome, and autism—a disorder character-
ized by "deviant reciprocal social interaction, delayed and aberrant communication skills, and a restricted repertoire of activities and interests" (Sadock &
Sadock, 2003, p. 1208). All of these disorders have been found to involve various problems in brain structure and/or function.

Engaging social neuroscience will lead to better understandings at the advocacy, the fundamental, the policy-making, and the day-to-day practice levels.
Yet mental health professionals encountering social neuroscience should not
request a menu of what to do and how to do it; they should be open to the
uncomfortable, the unfamiliar, and the less-than-certain.

Book Contents

Themes

This book has two main themes: (1) presentation of selected neuroscience
research findings in areas critical to social work and other human service professions, specifying why this knowledge is important for practicing clinicians
and indicating how these findings can influence the development of neuroscience; and (2) use of the transactional model as the conceptual framework
for incorporating neuroscientific knowledge into clinical practice.

Chapter-by-Chapter Outline

Chapter 1: Linking to the Neuroscientific Revolution

*Why should social workers and other human service professionals embrace the
missing link?* Linkage with social neuroscience is recommended. Neuroscience
and social neuroscience are outlined. Reasons for linking with the
neuroscientific revolution are discussed, and four levels of linkage with social
neuroscience are indicated.

Chapter 2: A Tour of the Brain

*What brain basics should a social worker know when beginning to engage in
neuroscience?* Selected characteristics, functions, and "geographical" features
are discussed.

Chapter 3: Neuroscience as Link: Transactional Model

*How can social work and other human service disciplines best understand
and contribute to the research findings of the neurosciences?* Enter the transactional model, which provides the conceptual framework for using this

new neuroscientific knowledge in social work and other disciplines. While we must be knowledgeable about the latest research findings from the neurosciences, I argue that biology alone is not destiny, and that we err if we get caught up in the biological determinism that findings from the "Decade of the Brain" compel us toward. The Transactional Model can serve as the framework for understanding and applying the latest neuroscience research findings to practice situations and for social work contributing to the development of social neuroscience.

Chapter 4: Linking to Social Work: Attaching and Bonding

How can neuroscientific research help in improving the understanding of attachment theory and human bonding in general? Social workers have historically worked with persons who experience environmental deprivations as well as serious emotional and psychiatric problems. As suggested earlier, we, and other mental health professionals, have recently been finding that clients have more intransigent and multiple problems and diagnoses. I suggest that recent neuroscience research provides some of the biological information that is necessary for understanding the etiology of these problems and how to intervene. It also presents us with the challenge of complexity in understanding human bonding in general.

Chapter 5: Linking to Social Work: Trauma

What is the relevance of neurobiological findings to work with children and adults who have been traumatized? To increase their reliance on science-based explanations, social workers should study trauma in the light of three main understandings. First, social workers should examine trauma within a neurodevelopmental perspective, seeking explanations in terms of the growth and functioning of the brain. Second, they should recognize that the biological is important but not "the" decisive determinant, as can be illustrated by considering the significance of a social or other dimension like that of the caretaker in childhood. Third, the social worker has an advocacy role, especially in identifying and arguing for the kind of neuroscientific research questions that he or she considers most relevant to the challenge of living.

Chapter 6: Linking to Social Work: Psychotherapy

How does neuroscience research fit or clash with psychotherapy? Neuroscience promises to transform both psychotherapeutic understandings and the practice of psychotherapy; it promises to enrich understanding and practice in clinical social work. Matters of understanding and of practice are considered. The first section discusses understanding, beginning with the dualism of mind and brain, the neurobiology of psychotherapy, and the relevance to clinical social work. For example, it is indicated why understanding will be deepened over time as the artificial and counterproductive character of the distinction between mind and brain is increasingly recognized in terms of treating mental illness. The second section examines promising neurobiological models for psychotherapeutic practice that use neuroscience results in terms of neural growth and integration; and results are demonstrated for such conditions as PTSD. It illustrates the practice significance of recognizing neural substrates of psychotherapeutic change. It discusses the practice relevance of the therapeutic relationship in terms of mirror neurons. Practice comments are illustrated with four case studies. The third section invites social work to embrace the opportunities proactively and realistically.

Chapter 7: Linking to Social Work: Medications and Drugs

How can neuroscience research help social workers and others intervene with persons who take prescribed psychotropic medications and those who are drug dependent and drug abusing?

During the past quarter century, we have seen the emergence of many new psychotropic medications, some of which have a more benign side effect profile than the older drugs. Since the early 1990s, it has been observed that there exist ethnic and individual differences in drug response; but as a result of the findings of the Human Genome Project, we now have some hard data to corroborate and explain these observations. This chapter reviews the main findings of this developing research, so that social workers and other human service professionals can become knowledgeable about differing medication response among African Americans, Asians, Hispanics, and women. Because we work with persons from these different ethnic and gender groups who use psychotropics, it behooves us to know about these differences so that we can facilitate medication management activities

In the second section, the focus is on the brain's pleasure circuit (the mesolimbic dopamine pathway) and its relationship to drugs of abuse. Enter neuroscience research to describe the processes of drug addiction, craving, and tolerance. Although the biological basis of drug use has become more widely accepted, there remains much stigma. To help lift the stigma, while providing more accurate knowledge, social workers and other practitioners need a better appreciation of what actually happens biologically when a person ingests a substance, why the substance use begins, and why it is so difficult to stop. This chapter also speaks to why substance use is such a challenging problem in our society. The transactional model is revisited, with specific application to medications that help and drugs that hurt.

Turn now to a tour of the brain.

2

Tour of the Brain

Let's go on a preliminary tour of the brain! Such a tour can be compared with travel to a foreign place. Like many foreign tours, a brain tour can be expected to be mainly about the complex and the unfamiliar.

Consider the incredible complexity of the typical human brain. It weighs about 3 lbs. and is a spongy mass of fatty tissue, the size of a coconut, and has "the consistency of an overripe peach" (Wylie & Simon, n.d.). It is implicated in controlling all bodily and all mental processes, including all learning and remembering, all feeling and thinking, and all behavior. The human brain contains some 100 billion neurons, and each neuron has from 10 to 100,000 synaptic connections. Neurons are interconnected into networks, with chemical and electrical communication systems. A single neuron can have thousands of receptor stations for the chemical neurotransmitters, and each neuron conducts electrical signals, enabling it to receive signals from thousands of cells within a millisecond. Many neuroscientists report that there are multineuronal functional units and that processes such as thinking and feelings arise from the integrated action of many neurons.

Brain tours are like travels to foreign lands, in that they are so exciting, so wondrous, and sometimes even anxiety provoking. One never can know exactly what it will be like. By the end of the chapter, the reader will know some basic characteristics of the brain as a whole and the ways that some functions are carried out by the brain (e.g., the ways that the brain remembers, learns, feels, and knows itself). Also of importance is knowing some geographical features of the brain (i.e., some main parts, such as the cerebral cortex and the amygdala; see Figure 2.1).

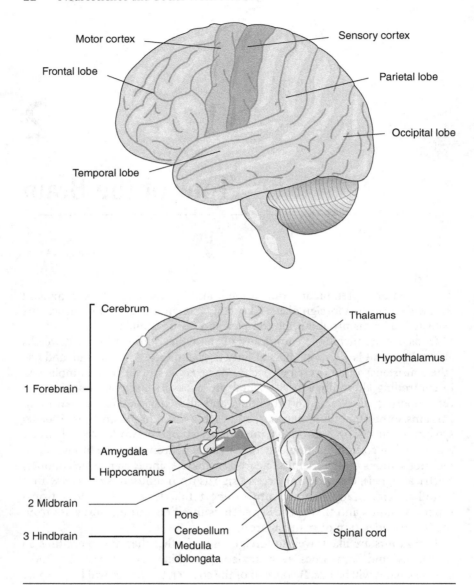

Figure 2.1 Brain Structure

Selected Characteristics

We start our tour of the brain with 10 introductory characteristics, which will help to deepen our understanding of this very complex foreign land and make for a marvelous journey.

First, brain-world is a fresh and valuable world. Valuable are the social neuroscience explanations about the subjects discussed in chapters 3 through 7, such as attachment, trauma, psychotherapy, psychotropic medications, and drugs of abuse. Neuroscience has the capability of changing our basic perceptions of ourselves and of the world. As one example, consider the emotional brain. A neuroscientific view is that we are emotional beings who think, rather than thinking beings who have emotions (LeDoux, 1996). Barring brain injury or malformation, a human nonemotional moment is a fiction. Also, there are views about the brain's sensory systems being narcissistic (e.g., see Atkins, 1996) and about where in the brain lying occurs; for instance, the anterior cingulate gyrus (e.g., see Tancredi, 2005).

Second, the brain carries out many actions automatically and below the level of conscious control (as discussed in chapter 5). Sometimes this leads to regrettable results (e.g., when one mistakes an automatic action for intuition that is always right). Yet most of the time, this process is useful (e.g., to provide immediate action needed for survival, or to provide brain time for more interesting dilemmas than "which hand shall I use to open the door?"; see Bear et al., 2007, pp. 564-583).

As an example, consider fear alarms implicated by encountering dangerous animals (e.g., when one is walking through underbrush and glimpses a partially obscured animal). Two neural pathways for fear alarms are activated (see LeDoux, 1996). One pathway leads from the thalamus to the amygdala. On seeing the animal, the emotional stimulus arrives at the brain's thalamus, and instantly, the body freezes with fear. Another pathway leads milliseconds later through the sensory cortex to awareness. Deciding that the animal is indeed harmless, one can unfreeze.

Other examples of the brain acting automatically could be added from evolutionary psychology, which is a combination of evolutionary biology and cognitive psychology. These activities might include eating the right foods, forming alliances, helping children, reading other people's minds, or selecting mates, all performed in the interest of preserving the genes (Evans & Zarate, 1999; Pinker, 1997).

Third, automatic functions or actions (i.e., those that seem to "just happen") occur mainly in the occipital, parietal, and temporal lobes—back, top, and side. Conscious control actions occur mainly in the cerebral cortex (e.g., forebrain—the front; Restak, 2006).

Fourth, the brain is plastic. For example, the brain is not all about genes. It's also about culture (Duncan, 2005; Wexler, 2006). Plasticity refers to the ever-changing nature of the brain due to the influence of environment. Embracing neuroscience does not mean that all is now basically biological.

To explain, senile decay starts when a brain is about 20 years old. But it is also important to remember that brain plasticity is lifelong. It's true that there are critical periods when the brain requires a specific experience to develop adequately. For example, most of us know that the best time to learn languages is before the preteen years. "Use it or lose it" is the brain's operating principle, even from the beginning. We are told that at 7 months of age, a typical child can hear sound differences in any language (he or she is a citizen of the world), and that at 11 months, a typical child has lost this ability (he or she has lost this world citizenship). It is also correct that brain functioning can be damaged (e.g., as in addiction, by altering the level of neurotransmitters) and it can be "hard-wired" (i.e., how connections of neurons and their synapses are joined with other neurons). Brain connections follow rules from the genes. For instance, Cynthia Kenyon reports increasing "the life span of tiny worms called Caenorhabdites elegans up to six times normal by suppressing a single gene" (Duncan, 2005, pp. 57-58). Yet the brain is continually changing in response to cultural and other inputs until the moment of death. (Even reading this book is changing your physical brain.) Like many other neuroscientists, Andreasen (2005) points out that we "are literally remaking our brains—who we are and how we think, with all our actions, reactions, perceptions, postures, and positions—every minute of the day and every day of the week and month and year of our entire lives" (p. 146).

We are not the mere "victims" of our biology; we can upgrade the functioning of our brains. For example, Nancy Andreasen (2005) recommends mental exercises to improve extraordinary creativity. She recommends that adults spend some time each day exploring an unfamiliar area of knowledge. She also advises spending some time each day practicing meditation or just thinking. The effect of activities on the brain is greatest in the frontal, temporal, and parietal regions. In addition, Andreasen advises that we practice observing and describing details intently.

Fifth, brain lesions—although regrettable and tragic—have value in helping us learn about "normal" brain functions. The classic example is that of the celebrated Phineas Gage, the railroad worker. (In 1848, an explosion sent an iron rod through Gage's skull, damaging the middle portions of his frontal cortex; his tragedy was instructive.) At the time, people who knew Gage could see that his personality was greatly changed, but in later years, it came to be understood that such frontal lobe injury results in serious emotional, motor, and cognitive changes. It may be that more is known about brain dysfunctions than functions.

Sixth, all brains are not the same. Yes, they are basically similar. But there are differences between groups (e.g., between female and male), within groups (e.g., within, as noted in chapter 1, the group of persons with schizophrenia), and between individuals.

For the neurobiology of the differences between female and male brains (such as the greater empathy among females), see Tancredi (2005). Female and male brains are very similar—more similar than dissimilar. But the typical female brain has a larger anterior commissure (connecting the temporal lobes) and a larger corpus callosum, especially the posterior part. (For discussion of diversity among those categorized as persons with schizophrenia, see Farmer & Pandurangi, 1997). Also, no two individuals are completely the same in regard to neural wiring, because brain plasticity makes for myriad interrelationships between genetic endowment and environmental input.

Seventh, human brains do differ from nonhuman brains. However, human and nonhuman brains are remarkably similar, and many of the explanations for human brains come from animal brain research. For example, Swanson (2003), noting that fewer than 0.1% of animal species incorporate the vertebrate body plan, states that in "the end, humans are really just a specialized vertebrate, and the organization of our nervous system—with its all-important brain—is simply a reflection of how the rest of our body is specialized relative to other vertebrate classes and species" (p. 44). Yet human and animal brains do differ significantly, for example, in the frontal and parietal lobes. (For a comparison of the brains of a human and a rat, see Bear et al., 2007.) Among the striking structural differences they list are the many convolutions on the surface of the human cerebrum—grooves (sulci) and bumps (gyri). "Clinical and experimental evidence indicate that the cortex is the seat of the uniquely human reasoning and cognition. Without cerebral cortex, a person would be blind, deaf, mute, and unable to initiate voluntary movement" (Bear et al., 2007, p. 194).

Eighth, we need to be cautious when applying concepts and metaphors from the familiar to the unfamiliar. That is, we should be cautious in applying concepts (e.g., from everyday experience to the brain, from one's home country to the foreign place we plan to visit). Many categories of thought that seem reasonable in cultural terms don't fit in brain terms.

On concepts, recall what was noted above about the emotional brain. Also see chapters 1 and 3, which discuss the example of the common distinction between thinking and emotion. It is said that distinction is hard for a brain to swallow. On the metaphor of the brain as a "computer, a solitary device with massive information-processing capabilities," Cacioppo, Visser, and Pickett (2006) comment that "At the dawn of the twenty-first century, this metaphor seems dated" and that it "is suddenly apparent that the teleceptors of the human brain have provided wireless broadband interconnectivity to humans for millennia" (p. xi).

Concepts are often changed by neuroscientific research. An example is the metaphor itself. Andrew Modell (2003) claims that metaphors—at the center of the imaginative—are not merely figures of speech. For him, they are neural features, the way that the brain yields meaning. Modell emphasizes that "the construction of meaning is very different from the processing of information" (p. 9). He discusses how metaphor is the brain's primary mode of understanding and remembering the world. He writes of metaphor in corporeal imagination in terms of transferring between dissimilar domains (e.g., as in synesthesia—"hearing" colors and "seeing" sounds).

Ninth, it is helpful to speak of a particular part (or parts) of the brain being responsible for particular functions. It's only useful, however, if we remember that it is a category mistake to speak of brain parts having functions: what happens at one neuroscientific level may not be a good description at other levels, and scientific research can produce fresh explanations over time. For instance, Berntson (2006), writes that "functions cannot really be localized at all, as they are . . . not properties of neuronal circuits or even the outputs of these circuits" (p. 2). A category error can occur when we mix facts, constructs, and theories from one domain (e.g., the psychological) with those of another domain (e.g., the biological domain) and find that the constructs do not match. As social workers, we can be prone to do this when our understanding of certain domains may be more limited than other domains.

Tenth, thou shalt not be deterred by forbidding terminology and by a "foreign" culture (as neuroscience is a foreign culture for a social worker or for any other nonneuroscientist).

For instance, it is not necessary to learn such details as the points of the compass to speaking about the parts of the brain: front, back, up, and down. Front, the nose end, is *anterior* or *rostral* (Latin for "beak"). The back end is *posterior* or *caudal* (Latin for "tail"). Up is *dorsal* (Latin for "back"). Down is *ventral* (Latin for "belly"). Other directional signs include *midsaggital plane* (plane splitting the brain into equal right and left halves), and *saggital plane* (any plane parallel to the midsaggital). Then there are *medial* (close to the midline), *lateral* (farther away from the midline), *ipsilateral* (on same side; e.g., left eye and left ear), and *contralateral* (on opposite sides; e.g., left ear and right ear).

At this point in the journey, the traveler might wonder if that is all there is to know about the brain and its workings. It seems necessary (in fact a no-brainer) to add another characteristic: *The neuroscientific revolution is in full swing!* A description of some specific functions of the brain will provide an elementary account of how the brain remembers, thinks, feels, and knows itself. We will see how even extremely elementary accounts can blow the mind. They seem to me poetic, sublime.

Selected Functions

Remembering

There are different kinds of memory. The kinds vary in type: declarative (or explicit memories of facts and events) and nondeclarative (or implicit memories of, for instance, skills and habits). They vary in terms of duration: short and long term; this is related because the short term can be consolidated and changed into long term. There is also working memory, just long enough to allow someone to remember and answer a question.

Different systems are involved in different types of memory. Long-term memories are ultimately stored in the neocortex. Declarative memory depends on a system involving the hippocampus and related segments, plus areas of the prefrontal cortex. Nondeclarative memory involves the striatum and the amygdala and cerebellum. Working memory depends on the prefrontal cortex and many other brain locations. The median temporal lobe, including the hippocampus, is implicated in converting from short-term to long-term memories. (For more about memory systems, see Bear et al., 2007.)

Memorizing includes changes in synapses between neurons—in the wiring of neurons. For more about related molecular and other processes involved in changing the synapses, see three Society for Neuroscience "Brain Briefings" (1997, 2000, 2004). These Brain Briefings are published monthly, summarize recent research regarding some items of interest concerning the brain, and are intended for a lay as well as scientific readership. One Brain Briefing is about a family of molecules, the cyclic amp-response element binding (CREB) protein implicated, for instance, in creating long-term memories (Society for Neuroscience, 1997). A second Brain Briefing discussed the role of insulin in memorizing (Society for Neuroscience, 1999). A third briefing reports on the chemical glutamate, involved in creating reactions that aid memory (Society for Neuroscience, 2004). Glutamate, a neurotransmitter, is also important for the development of long-term potentiation, which is discussed next, in relation to learning.

Learning

Surprise, surprise! There are different kinds of learning. There is nonassociative learning, which is open to all animals and humans and which is in response to a single type of stimulus (e.g., habituation and sensitization). Then there is associative learning, which requires a nervous system and forms associations between events (e.g., classical and instrumental conditioning). Classical conditioning was described by Pavlov, and instrumental or operant conditioning was made famous by B.F. Skinner. In the latter, the human or animal does something and learns from the positive or negative feedback resulting from that action.

No single brain structure or mechanism accounts for learning, acquiring new information, and so forth. Perhaps more useful for the tourist-to-be is to conceptualize learning as synaptic plasticity, the brain continually accommodating to the environment. Swanson (2003) reports that it is likely that the critical site for such plasticity is the cerebrum (i.e., cerebral hemisphere or "large brain"), rather than the cerebellum (i.e., "small brain"). He notes that the best way of studying the chemistry of synaptic plasticity is to use long-term potentiation (LTP), which has been studied in a number of brain locations. He concludes that the "bottom line is that there are many mechanisms for changing the strength of synapses with use. . . . These cellular mechanisms range from habituation and sensitization, through tetanic and posttetanic potentiation, to long-term potentiation and depression" (Swanson, 2003, p. 210). Synaptic plasticity and LTP were topics much discussed at the recent annual meeting of the Society for Neuroscience. LTP is the process by which new wiring occurs, and it describes how a neuronal response increases as a result of being stimulated; it helps explain the cellular and molecular changes that take place in the brain as a result of learning.

Feeling

The following are eight points that will prepare the potential tourist for "brain-world." They are eight themes that Joseph LeDoux (1996) describes in his book *The Emotional Brain*. (LeDoux is well known for his work on the brain mechanisms of emotions.) Then we turn to happiness, as discussed in a Society for Neuroscience (2000) Brain Briefing. The emotional brain consists mainly of the amygdala, the hippocampus, the anterior cingulate cortex, and the hypothalamus. These brain parts and their significance are further discussed in chapter 4.

First, there is "no such thing as the 'emotion' faculty and there is no single brain system dedicated to this phantom function" (LeDoux, 1996, p. 16). LeDoux explains that the word *emotion* does not refer to something the brain or mind really has or does. Rather, it is a label for something related to the brain and mind. He is supported in his contention about the nature of emotions by Antonio Damasio, a leading neuroscientist at the University of Iowa, who is well known for his research on the neurology of emotion, memory, and language. Damasio (2003) wants to reconstruct the word *feelings*, correcting the commonsensical and argues (as James-Lange did before; e.g., see Bear et al., 2007) that an emotional feeling is identical to the bodily sensations that express it and that emotions do not cause bodily symptoms but vice versa. Damasio claims that of "all the mental phenomena we can describe, feelings and their essential ingredients—pain and pleasure—are the least understood in biological and specifically neurobiological terms" (p. 3).

Second, brain systems reflect many levels of evolutionary history. It seems that "the neural organization of particular emotional behavioral systems—like the systems underlying fearful, sexual, or feeding behaviors—is pretty similar across species" (LeDoux, 1996, p. 17). Humans, as well as fish, amphibians, reptiles, birds, and other mammals have neuronal systems that allow for survival and procreation.

Third, when an animal has the capacity for conscious awareness, it can have conscious emotional feelings. Otherwise, the animal's brain pursues its survival goals unconsciously. LeDoux writes, "And absence of awareness is the rule of mental life, rather than the exception, throughout the animal kingdom" (p. 17). In other words, emotional responses develop out of the unconscious, and feelings do not need to be conscious to result in emotional behavior.

Fourth, conscious feelings are mere detours in studying emotions. For example, the fundamental mechanism of fear is the system that detects danger, not the emotion. We can easily be distracted by focusing solely on the feelings. There is much more to a feeling than what appears on the surface.

Fifth, understanding "emotions in the human brain is clearly an important quest, as most mental disorders are emotional disorders" (LeDoux, 1996, pp. 18-19). Because the emotional responses are generated by the same brain system in animals and people, and because research on the neural basis of emotions in humans is fraught with ethical and practical concerns, LeDoux concludes that there is great value in using animal studies to understand how emotions are generated in people.

Sixth, "states of consciousness occur when the system responsible for awareness becomes privy to the activity occurring in unconscious processing systems" (LeDoux, 1996, p. 19). Consciousness can be filled with facts and minutiae or powerful emotions. The emotions tend to take over and obliterate the mundane, whereas thoughts (which are not emotional) cannot easily displace the feelings.

Seventh, "emotions are things that happen to us rather than things we will to occur" (LeDoux, 1996, p. 19). In other words, emotions originate in the lower brain (i.e., amygdala) and are nonconscious. Le Doux also notes that as of now, humans have evolved to the point where the connections emanating from the lower brain and traveling to the higher cortical areas are stronger than those connections that proceed in the opposite direction (i.e., from the cognitive to the emotional systems). We see in chapter 7 how this is an important factor in psychotherapeutic interventions.

Eighth, when emotions happen, they "become powerful motivators of future behaviors" (LeDoux, 1996, p. 19). LeDoux notes that emotions propel us toward achievement but can also lead us into difficulties. They can help us to stay mentally healthy or, as in addictions and other mental illnesses, can reflect an emotional breakdown.

The Society for Neuroscience's (2000) Brain Briefing "Bliss and the Brain" associates happy feelings with the prefrontal cortex. It reports that "right side activation links to negative feelings, whereas left-side activation links to positive feelings." Positron emission tomography studies, which map the fear and anxiety circuit in human brains, also show increased blood flow in fear pathways of the brain (amygdala, hippocampus, thalamus, anterior cingulate, and inferior frontal regions), when people are shown very unpleasant images. When people were shown pleasant images, "higher" parts of the brain located in the cerebral cortex were activated (Andreasen, 2001).

Mirroring

Consider mirror neurons. Tancredi (2005) explains that mirror neurons "in humans involve a network which is formed by the temporal, occipital, and parietal visual areas, as well as two additional cortical regions that are predominantly motor" (p. 40). Mirror neurons make it possible for us to learn complex motor skills merely by watching others perform these same skills. They link visual and motor experiences; make possible implicit learning via imitation of what is seen, heard, and felt; and are thought to be involved in understanding the intentions of others.

Knowing Itself

Celebrate the frontal lobes as the seat of self-awareness, celebrate the prefrontal cortex as the center of understanding, and damn the torpedoes!

The torpedoes in this case include the confusion and disagreement about the nature of a self, not less than of self awareness, no less than of the neural correlates. They also include the fact that all these "functions"—remembering, learning, feeling, knowing oneself and others—interrelate; they are rough-and-ready conceptual categories, designed in preneuro times. There are divergences of view and more conversations and research studies to come. The torpedoes also include the genuine difficulties of this much-researched topic (e.g., see Feinberg & Keenan, 2005).

For the potential traveler, recognizing levels of awareness (how many levels compose a different question) is attractive. In their chapter titled "The Frontal Lobes and Self-Awareness," Stuss, Rosenblum, Malcolm, Christina, and Keenan (2005) describe four levels of awareness. The first is being conscious, as opposed to unconscious. The second involves processing the basic contents or knowledge of the world, and that is reported to implicate the more posterior cortical regions and the posterior motor areas. The third level, the concept developed from a patient with bilateral frontal lobe damage and mistaking his family for a new family, involves an appropriate sense of identity that implicates appropriate sameness and continuity. The fourth level of awareness is "one that views all information in light of a personal history, from the past and projecting into the future" (p. 53). Stuss et al. make the point that this is both a bottom-up and a top-down model; the higher levels affect the lower and vice versa.

Underlining how brain functions are interrelated is the attractive idea of the autobiographical self: A self-aware person, the traveler might think, is surely a person capable of knowing his or her own story. In their chapter on autobiographical disorders, Fujiwara and Markowitsch (2005) speak of the complexity of autobiographical memory:

> This complexity is embodied in the large network of activated brain regions during autobiographical memory retrieval, which involves core memory regions (the hippocampal formation), areas of self-related processing (medial prefrontal cortex), and those of sensory-emotional integration (posterior association cortex and posterior cingulate gyrus) . . . effective recollection of autobiographical memories requires all these areas. (p. 75)

Fujiwara and Markowitsch also note that autobiographical capability rarely corresponds to circumscribed areas of the brain.

Brain functions do appear to be very interrelated! As we continue our travel to this new brain world, let's focus on a few geographical (i.e., structural) features. This would be akin to traveling overseas and knowing the locations of cities such as London or Shanghai.

Selected Geographical Features

It is helpful to remember that most brain parts come in twos, one for each side of the brain (right hemisphere and left hemisphere). So there are two amygdalae, two hippocampi, and so on. The brain structures are listed in alphabetical order (see Figure 2.2).

Amygdala: Located in the forebrain—in the anterior temporal (side, temple) lobe. It's an almond-shaped nucleus and an important component of the limbic system. It is involved in emotional learning, especially when fear is involved.

Anterior Cingulate Gyrus: Involved with maternal behavior, nursing, and play; helps us to focus our attention, involved with emotional response and part of the extended limbic system; drugs of abuse impair this part of the brain.

Basal Ganglia: This is a cluster of neurons, which include the caudate nucleus, putamen, globus pallidus, and substantia nigra. Located deep within the brain, this cluster plays an important role in movement.

Brainstem: Major route by which the forebrain sends information to and receives information from the spinal cord and peripheral nerves; it controls respiration and regulation of heart rhythms.

Broca's Area: Located in the frontal lobe of the left hemisphere; important for the production of speech.

Central Nervous System: Brain and spinal cord.

Central Sulcus: A sulcus is a groove. The central sulcus divides the parietal lobe and the frontal lobe—a kind of Grand Canyon between the middle and the front of the brain.

Cerebellum: At the roof of the hind brain, or what looks to be at the nape of the neck. It is a movement control center and recently found to be also involved in cognitive and emotional functions.

Cerebral Cortex: This is the outermost layer of the cerebral hemispheres and is divided into four lobes (occipital, temporal, parietal, and frontal). It is responsible for all forms of conscious experience, including perception, emotion, thinking, and planning.

Cerebral Hemispheres: These are the two sides of the cerebral cortex. The left hemisphere (for right-handed people) is specialized for speech, language, writing,

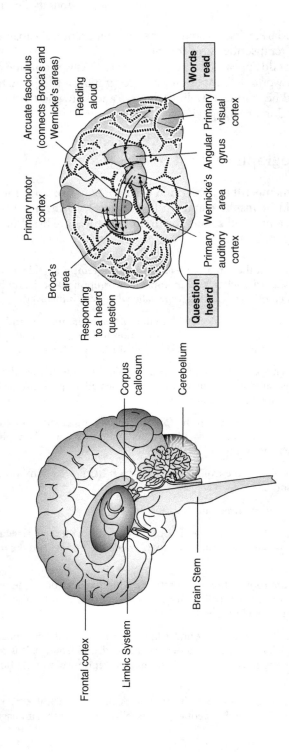

Figure 2.2 Brain Structures

and calculation, and is especially involved with the details of a situation. The right hemisphere (for right-handed people) is specialized for face recognition, spatial abilities, nonverbal communication, and processing emotional experience.

Corpus Callosum: A commissure is any set of axons that connects one side of the brain with the other. This is the "mother" of all commissures, the great connector of the two cerebral hemispheres. It begins to develop toward the end of the first year of life and eventually makes possible cognitive and emotional integration.

Forebrain: This includes the cerebral cortex and basal ganglia, which are credited with the highest intellectual functions.

Fornix: A bundle of axons (i.e., extension of neuron by which the cell sends information to other cells), which conducts nerve impulses and action potentials (when a neuron is activated and changes its electrical charge from negative to positive). It starts in the hippocampal formation, loops around the thalamus, and ends in the diencephalon, which is known as the "between brain" and includes the thalamus and hypothalamus.

Frontal Lobe: One of the four parts of the cerebral cortex, it is located in front of the central sulcus (see above). The other three parts are the parietal, temporal, and occipital lobes. The frontal lobe is involved in controlling movement, planning and coordinating behavior, and abstract reasoning (i.e., executive functions of the brain).

Hippocampus: It is shaped like a sea horse and is located in the temporal lobe, which is part of the limbic system. It plays a part in learning, memory, and emotion.

Hypothalamus: It has many nuclei, with different functions including involvement in regulating internal organs, monitoring information from the autonomic nervous system, controlling the pituitary gland, and regulating appetite and sleep.

Limbic System: This is a group of brain structures, including the amygdala, hippocampus, septum, basal ganglia, and others. It is involved in emotion, learning, and memory and regulates basic body functions such as thirst, hunger, and sex drive.

Locus Coeruleus: Center for norepinephrine cells; it releases noradrenalin to the amygdalae and hippocampi and is therefore involved in the stress response.

Midbrain: This is located in the anterior (front) segment of the brainstem. It is involved in regulating respiration, perception of pain, heart rate, and movement.

Neocortex: This is the newer, more highly evolved cortical area, also called the cerebral cortex. It is found only in mammals.

Nucleus Accumbens: Located in the basal ganglia part of the brain; it is involved in reward expectation and emotional modulation.

Occipital Lobe: One of the four parts of the cerebral cortex (see frontal lobe). It is implicated in processing visual data.

Orbitofrontal Cortex: Located right behind the eyes, it is involved in cognitive processes such as decision making; it is also involved with emotions and sense of reward and punishment.

Parietal Lobe: One of four parts of the cerebral cortex (see frontal lobe). It is involved in sensory processes, attention, and language.

Peripheral Nervous System: This is the nervous system other than brain and spinal cord (i.e., the autonomic and somatic nervous systems). These systems involve communication with the sense organs and glands and thus involve the whole body.

Pituitary Gland: An endocrine organ closely linked with and controlled by the hypothalamus. It secretes hormones that regulate the activity of other endocrine organs in the body.

Pons: Part of the hindbrain and called "the bridge," because it connects the cerebrum with the spinal cord and cerebellum. It controls respiration and heart rhythms and is the major route for the forebrain to transmit and receive information to and from the spinal cord and autonomic nervous system.

Synapse: A gap between two neurons; it functions as the site of information transfer from one neuron to another.

Temporal Lobe: One of the four major divisions of the cerebral cortex. It is implicated in speech and in auditory and visual perception.

Thalamus: Two egg-shaped, walnut-sized masses of nerve tissue located deep within the brain. It is the information relay station, which serves as a central switchboard and is key in filtering out unimportant information and sending on signals that require action.

Ventricles: Large spaces filled with cerebrospinal fluid; three are located in the brain and one in the brainstem.

Wernicke's Area: The brain region responsible for language comprehension and production of meaningful speech.

Thus ends our preliminary tour of the brain. As our travels to brain world continue, let's now turn to the Transactional Model.

3

Neuroscience as Link

Transactional Model

Neuroscience is a missing link that can upgrade, or even downgrade, social work and other helping disciplines. The linking will upgrade social work if neuroscience is understood within a framework that includes what I describe as the transactional model. It can downgrade, to varying extents, if neuroscientific results are not interpreted in an appropriate fashion.

Twin and opposing mistakes are overenthusiasm and underenthusiasm. To put it another way, it is like being between Scylla and Charybdis, or a rock and a hard place. On one hand, it is a mistake to overenthusiastically swing from a situation where the biological is neglected to a situation where the biological is overemphasized. It is likewise erroneous to fail to recognize the limits of positivism. On the other hand, it is also a mistake to be underenthusiastic about the insights made possible by advances in the neurosciences. Such opposing mistakes can result from simple misunderstandings (e.g., when some parents of children with schizophrenia have welcomed scientific or biological evidence that makes their children's affliction less unbearable but neglect the nonbiological understandings that are also available). More fundamentally, such mistakes occur when there is no appropriate conceptual framework—a framework like that provided by the transactional model.

The term *missing link* can be seen as symbolic of such difficulty. It is misleading, for instance, if it is assumed that in evolutionary theory there has to be a sole missing link. Similarly, it is misleading in biologically informed social work to assume that the biological is the sole cause. The missing link has excited both overenthusiasm and underenthusiasm. On the one hand, embracing the missing link can excite a sort of missionary zeal. On the other hand, the

35

negative fear that surrounds the idea of evolution—that is symbolized by the missing link—hardly needs illustration. Similarly, the neuroscientific revolution can evoke fears among social workers and other helping professionals as it represents challenges to entrenched ideas and practices. Some human service practitioners have given only lip service to the biological because they fear to infringe on traditional thinking and practice.

In the first two subsections, this chapter underscores aspects of the overenthusiasm and the underenthusiasm for the biological, for neuroscience talk. Then it describes and analyzes a transactional framework, which is recommended for social work to engage the missing link of neuroscience. This was first written about in relation to the teaching of human behavior in the advanced clinical curriculum of master of social work programs (Farmer, 1999). In that context, the transactional model was used to address the problem of underconcentration in our understanding of the biological aspects of human behavior. In the present context, the model is used to focus our data collection on all of the relevant domains (i.e., biological, psychological, social, spiritual, and challenge in living) for informing clinical interventions.

Overenthusiasm

"The Pleasure Neuron: Luxury may be habit-forming and we have the MRIs (magnetic resonance imaging) to prove it." Illustrating how brain talk has become part of enthusiastic everyday talk, this advertisement for a brand of car caught my eye ("The Pleasure Neuron," 2005). The heroine of the advertisement is a neurosurgeon, and her weapon is neuroscience. The advertisement for the high-priced car, a Lincoln, touts the car's audio system as inducing "a harmonious brain state, no matter how snarled the traffic." Happy brain talk! The neurosurgeon-owner talks about how she loves the car and how the *nucleus accumbens* is a part of the brain that is important to pleasure. This particular brand of car, the neurosurgeon explains, "provides stimulation for all the senses" (p. 2). It's stimulation for the brain, because, as she explains, the brain is the repository of all that we see, feel, think, and experience; the car is brainy.

Brain talk and brain terms are being used in our everyday lives. They have become acceptable, at least in this one advertisement for readers of the *New York Times*. Neuroscience is being used to sell luxury cars. Brain talk is now an integral part of our culture. To provide the most up-to-date and effective interventions for our clients, we need to incorporate research findings from the neurosciences into our knowledge base. As human service professionals, we also need to advocate for those particular neuroscience research questions, rather than others, that will yield understandings useful for our clients.

Although enthusiasm is desirable, overenthusiasm in brain talk can be counterproductive; however, I want to draw attention to two kinds of overenthusiasm that I think also underlies the rhetoric in the advertisement for the high-priced car. The first is where brain talk is taken to stand in a privileged epistemological position precisely because it is science talk and the limitations of positivism are not recognized. To put it another way, a true scientific proposition is understood as having a greater claim on my assent than a true nonscientific proposition, because I have more assurance that the scientific proposition is true (a scientific fact vs. a nonscientific fact). Yet there is a failure to appreciate the consensus in the immense and well-known literature on the nature, strengths, and limitations of positivism (e.g., Boyd & Gasper, 1993). The consensus is that positivist disciplines, like those involved in neuroscience, yield explanations rather than understandings; they produce causes rather than reasons. Positivism is highly successful and useful precisely because it is designed to exclude classes of understanding, like meaning. It suggests the desirability of social workers preparing themselves with a basic understanding of philosophy of science so that they can manage this kind of overenthusiasm (see Diesing, 1991).

The second kind of overenthusiasm (which I discuss at greater length) is where biological causation is understood to be total. In other words, overenthusiasm falls into the exaggeration of biological determinism. This kind of overenthusiasm is also connected with a lack of sophistication, symbolized by the rhetoric in the advertisement for the car. Social workers are used to such simplification when we hear clients saying things like, "I have schizophrenia; it's a brain disease," or "I'm depressed; it's all in my brain." How about the clinician who encounters a client who carries a diagnosis of schizophrenia and immediately assesses the person as having a brain disease? Yes, these statements are true in part, but they do not fully capture the etiology of either of these illnesses. How often do we encounter a person and think, "I wonder what kind of parents they had," or "What kind of trauma experience led them to do that?" or "Where did they get such a personality?" Each of these scenarios comes down on one side or the other of the nature and nurture dichotomy.

Let me say more about the second kind of overenthusiasm, speaking in terms of the nature versus nurture debate. For many years, those interested in human behavior have tended to form themselves into two camps of adherents, those who believe that all human behavior is the result of biology and those who argue that all behavior is the result of the sociocultural environment (the biological vs. the social sciences). There is ongoing debate on this topic. With the explosion of neuroscientific research during the past 20 years, many think that we have now entered an era of biological determinism. In other words, it is supposed that the proliferation of brain research places us exclusively on the side of nature, with little respect for the power of nurture.

Let us express the argument in terms of genes and behavior. Do people's genes make them behave in a particular way? Can people control their behavior? These fundamental questions are raised by the ELSI program of the Human Genome Project (1990-2003), noted in chapter 1. These questions are raised under the ELSI's heading of "conceptual and philosophical implications about human responsibility, free will vs. genetic determinism, and concepts of health and disease" (U.S. Department of Energy, n.d.).

It is accurate to say that brain connections follow rules from the genes. For example, Richard Dawkins discusses the "selfish gene" (Dawkins, 1976). It is an understanding of social behavior and evolution, associated with thinkers such as George Williams (1966) and William Hamilton (1964). The basic idea of the selfish gene is that individuals do not always take actions for the benefit of other individuals. Rather, they pursue actions at the biological level for the good of their genes. Sometimes the good of the individual and the good of the genes coincide, but not always. As Dawkins puts it, "We are survival machines—robot vehicles blindly programmed to preserve the selfish molecules known as genes" (p. 21). Later, Haig (1993) indicated that the contest on behalf of genes can occur even in the human womb, as mother and fetus (whose genes are not identical) can struggle over blood sugar. He reports that the fetus secretes human placental lactogen (hPL) that blocks the effects of the mother's insulin. Clearly, genes are important. The argument is unaffected by the reality that behaviors involve multiple genes and that there are problems in defining specific behaviors. But is that the end of the argument?

Siegel (1999) is one who argues that the term *biological determinism* is mistaken and that the opposite is much closer to the truth. He believes that the brain's structure and function are shaped by one's interactions with the environment, and therefore, nature and nurture is a false dichotomy. Strohman (2003), a molecular and cell biologist, also is concerned about the overemphasis placed on biology. He notes that genes alone cause only about 2% of the total disease load in human beings (e.g., diseases such as sickle cell anemia and Duchenne muscular dystrophy), whereas 98% of human diseases (e.g., cancer and heart disease) are polygenic, multifactorial diseases. Strohman refers to such common diseases as "diseases of civilization." In these 98% of diseases, genes may be necessary causes, but they are not sufficient causes. Because polygenic traits and diseases are not part of a linear process (i.e., a single gene or a set of genes leading to a single disease) and there are strong environmental interactions, Strohman argues for a move from genetic reductionism to epigenetic regulation.

Most psychosocial practitioners will recognize the term *epigenetic* from the work of Erik Erikson (1950) who borrowed the term from embryology. Erikson used the epigenetic principle to describe a child's development as occurring in sequential stages, each of which had to be satisfactorily resolved for development to proceed normally. Strohman (2003) describes the activity of genes as following an epigenetic path, which involves gene–gene interactions, gene–protein interactions, and all of these interacting with environmental signals. Other researchers also believe that talk of nature versus nurture is unhelpful. What is more useful is to focus on the epigenetic nature of development, where biology and experience work together to enhance adaptation (Gottesman & Hanson, 2005; Mascolo & Fischer, 2004). Although it is true that human service professionals need to be knowledgeable about the latest research findings from the neurosciences, it also needs to be said that biology alone is not destiny, and we err if we get caught up in the biological determinism that Strohman (2003), Siegel (1999), and others have warned against.

Some researchers support the doctrine of multilevel analysis in the study of mental and behavioral phenomena (e.g., Cacioppo & Berntson, 1992). They conceptualize the social and the neurological perspectives as two ends of a continuum. Basic research needs to cut across all these levels to integrate them and prevent reductionistic analyses. So, for example, depression, schizophrenia, juvenile delinquency, and child and spousal abuse are social and neurophysiological phenomena. Bruce Wexler (2006) is among those who would view such a continuum model as understating the case. His view is that the "relationship between the individual and the environment is so extensive that it almost overstates the distinction between the two to speak of a relationship at all. The body is in a constant process of gas, fluid, and nutrient exchange with the environment, and the defining feature of each body organ is its role in these processes. The brain and its sensory processes are no exception" (p. 39).

There is also the reality of brain plasticity, to which we will return later. The brain is continually changing in response to cultural and other inputs until the moment of death. Like many other neuroscientists, Nancy Andreasen (2005) points out that, as the reader reads, the reader's brain is changing. I am remaking my brain as I write.

We have used the term *environment* in several contexts, and perhaps a clearer understanding of this complex term will enhance our discussion. Environment denotes the total surrounding, everything that is external to the person but has actually become a part of the person. For example, family members, neighbors, and other community components such as schools are part of the environment for a particular person. There is also the distinction between what is inherited (nature) and everything else (nurture; i.e., the environmental).

In the late nineteenth century, Sir Francis Galton, the father of twin research, introduced the idea that the study of twins could help us distinguish nature from nurture or the difference between what is inherited and what comes from the environment. In their landmark study on the biological roots of schizophrenia and manic-depressive disorder, Torrey, Bowler, Taylor, and Gottesman (1994) refer to Galton and his contributions to the present-day study of mental illness. They also point out the importance of the nongenetic and environmental factors that appear to originate outside the person but can become a part of him or her. For example, genetic theories of schizophrenia have included the study of such prenatal and perinatal environmental influences as viruses, birth trauma, infections, anoxia, and stress. In their own research, Torrey et al. found a possible link between pestiviruses and schizophrenia, and obstetrical complications were an important etiological factor in at least 30% of the twins they studied who had schizophrenia. In these situations, the virus would be considered an environmental factor, but it is also clearly a biological and nongenetic factor. Obstetrical complications (e.g., low birth weight, breech birth, use of forceps, and toxemia) are also biological events that are nongenetic and environmental risk factors for schizophrenia. Therefore, in talking about the environment and its contribution to illness, we may be referring to early exposure to a toxin and/or physical trauma at key development periods, which then interacts with biological factors to result in various anomalies (Edward H. Taylor, personal communication, January 18, 2008).

The idea that environment may not be solely a social factor may be difficult for social workers and other human service professionals to consider, but it is important that we do so. When speaking in social terms, and related to mental illness, it may be easy for the reader to assume that we are saying that environment (e.g., parents) can be the causative factor for illnesses such as autism, schizophrenia, and bipolar disorder. This is not our intent, because it is clear to this writer that such illnesses have a clear biological etiology.

Recent studies in the neurosciences point to human development and behavior as being the result of a very complex interplay between nature and nurture. So whether we are describing normal processes and outcomes or abnormal manifestations (i.e., mental illnesses and other maladaptations), it is not only simplistic but also egregiously inadequate to dichotomize this issue. It is preferable to study the interaction between nature and nurture (e.g., the interaction of gene and environment; Meaney, 2004; Siegel, 1999). The overenthusiasm of biological reductionism is, in my view, unwarranted.

Underenthusiasm

Underenthusiasm for the neuroscientific revolution is as unwarranted and as harmful as overenthusiasm. The fact is that many of the findings from neuroscience are indeed worthy of enthusiasm, and I want to illustrate this with the briefest sketch of thinking about the development of the brain itself. On the question of underenthusiasm, let's acknowledge that in the nature versus nurture debate (just mentioned), some individuals have already decided which of the two positions they favor. For example, there are studies that measure the extent to which mental health professionals assign etiological responsibility (for emotional and behavioral disorders) to parents (Johnson et al., 2000; Rubin, Cardenas, Warren, Pike, & Wambach, 1998). Many professionals still favor the nurture side of the dichotomy, which influences their work with clients and their families. For example, although we now know that the pleasure circuit in the brain (the mesolimbic dopamine pathway) and genetic inheritance play a major role in the development of drug dependencies, some human service professionals continue to blame the drug-dependent individual for their illness. I take this to be a manifestation of underenthusiasm for the findings of the brain sciences.

As an example of neuroscientific knowledge worthy of enthusiasm, turn to a sketch (though leaving out a mass of details) of the development of the brain. Research from the neurosciences helps us to appreciate that the brain is an organ that continually grows. Until recently, the brain was conceptualized as being static once it reached maturity. This led to pessimism related to brain defects and damage. However, as a result of the neuroscience research of the past 25 years (and as mentioned earlier), we now know more about the brain's plasticity (i.e., ability to change based on experience) and that it continues to grow and develop (and decline) throughout the life course. This is important for social workers to know because it brings more realistic understanding of the results of various brain insults, an appreciation for rehabilitation efforts, and understanding about what the brain needs at various times to develop in a healthy manner. For example, there have been major changes in the way stroke victims can be rehabilitated. In the past, a 75-year-old person who had a stroke that affected the language center of the brain might be left untreated poststroke (based on ageism and the faulty belief that after early adulthood, the brain no longer can grow). Nowadays, such a person is offered aggressive remedial physical therapy, which can improve language capacity.

The brain develops in a hierarchical fashion, beginning with the more primitive regions (brainstem and diencephalon) during gestation and progressing to the more complex limbic and cortical areas during childhood. Within the first trimester after conception, the DNA, which is encoded within each cell, transmits the message for some cells to become neurons. These neurons begin to form axons and dendrites; they migrate to the appropriate neural tube location, which eventually becomes the brain, and they develop connections with each other. The actual connecting points are called synapses, and these continue to form during fetal life, a process called synaptogenesis. Also during this time, neurotransmitters such as dopamine, serotonin, and norepenephrine are manufactured, and these chemical messengers enhance communication between neurons (see Figure 3.1). By 6 months of gestational age, the traditional wisdom is that the central nervous system of the fetus has attained its total number of neurons (Shonkoff & Meisels, 2000), though the process of differentiation continues.

Each person's genetic makeup provides a template for future growth; as noted in chapter 1, there are approximately 30,000 human genes, and one third are expressed in the brain. As the brain grows, it proceeds through critical periods of development (when a specific brain region is organizing and requires a specific experience at that exact time) and through sensitive periods (when

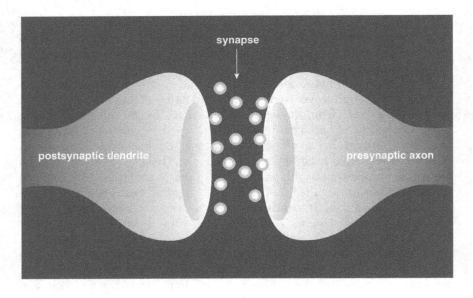

Figure 3.1   Neurons Firing

certain experiences are most sensitive for the brain). During the last trimester of prenatal development, a major growth spurt occurs in brain tissue. This is considered to be a critical period in brain development, and at this time, it is especially important for the fetus to receive an adequate intake of protein and calories. If not, it is reported that the number of brain cells can be reduced by as much as 40%.

At birth, the human infant's brain weighs only 25% of its full adult weight. By the age of 2 years, the brain has reached 75% of its final weight (Davies, 2004). This huge growth spurt during the first 2 years of life represents increasing complexity of the central nervous system (brain and spinal cord), which is accompanied by increasing amounts of synaptogenesis and myelination of axons (the myelin sheath insulates the axon and allows for electrical signals to travel about 100 times faster). The immediate postnatal period is one of those critical periods for brain development, during which a tremendous amount of linking and wiring occurs between brain systems. For example, at birth, the brainstem (which regulates heart rate, blood pressure, and breathing) needs to be functioning for the infant to survive. Postnatally, this system begins a process of linking with the frontal cortex (where cognitive and executive functions develop) and the limbic system (the seat of attachment, affect regulation, and emotion).

At 3 months of age, more brain regions become active, and the infant can now track visually and reach for and grab objects nearby. At 8 months of age, the frontal cortex has become active and allows the infant to think about danger. This is represented by the "stranger anxiety," which occurs among children in all cultures. At about 12 months of age, the young child is able to walk, which is a direct result of the myelination of spinal cord nerve pathways. This is a good exemplar for how knowledge about brain development is crucial for parents and other caretakers. No matter how much prodding we might do, the child is unable to walk until certain physiological processes have developed.

During this first year of life, and as discussed in chapter 4, it is reported that an important aspect of brain development is the quality of interactions between the child and the caregiver. When the interactions are mainly positive, the neural circuits involved become associated with positive affective quality. But when child–caregiver interactions are negative, the neural circuits become charged with negative affects (Shapiro & Applegate, 2000). Again, we can see how an underenthusiasm for the contributions of brain science impacts our understanding of the quality of neural circuits that develop and the ensuing quality of interpersonal relationships. This may provide an explanation for what happens to some persons who seem destined to have more negative than positive interactions with other people.

A crucial consideration is that all of the brain systems develop and store information in what is referred to as a "use-dependent" manner. In other words, neurons and synapses that are stimulated grow thicker dendrites and spines, and that strengthens the neuronal connections that are used. Synapses are created based on repetition of actions, thoughts, and behaviors (Perry, 2000). At the same time, synapses that are not used are "pruned away"—the "use it or lose it" principle. These processes are shaped by one's genetic encoding in interaction with experience, which determines how neurons are to grow, make connections, and die (Siegel, 1999).

These are examples of the brain's plasticity, especially active in the early years but continuing throughout life. The brain's receptivity to environmental influences (plasticity) makes it open to the joys of positive stimuli. Unfortunately, it also makes it vulnerable to negative stimuli such as neglect, abuse, trauma, and malnutrition (Davies, 2004). This is discussed further in chapter 5.

Recognizing such contributions from neuroscience, isn't there sufficient reason for social workers and others to be justifiably enthused about the research that brings such knowledge? We have argued here that an all-out embracing of recent neuroscience findings, or a total lack of appreciation for such findings, will impair progress in achieving new understandings and solutions to the challenges of human behavior.

The Model

A transactional model (Farmer, 1999) can provide a conceptual map for understanding and for applying human behavior knowledge, including neuroscientific data, for the benefit of our clients. The model provides an approach for understanding the dynamic interrelationships between the biological, the psychological, the social, the spiritual, and the challenge in living. This section describes each component or each *holon* (a term described later), and it discusses how they interact with each other to provide the necessary assessment data that is required in day-to-day practice situations.

Components

Four components make up the model. The biological domain includes what we have discussed as neuroscience; it includes genetic processes, the brain and spinal cord (Central Nervous System), and other biological systems of the body (e.g., the endocrine, digestive, respiratory, cardiovascular, and immune systems). The psychological domain consists of behavior and mental processes that involve cognition, emotion, and motivation. This includes intrapsychic processes, cognitive processes, defense mechanisms, and coping strategies. The social domain refers to interpersonal and family relationships, societal processes, and political and cultural issues and events (e.g., cultural or ethnic identity). The spiritual domain involves belief behaviors and patterns that are used to understand life's meaning, purpose, and one's connection to others and the world. These beliefs can be used in the service of coping and adaptation (Sermabeikian, 1994).

Two caveats should be noted. One is about spirituality. The role of religion and spirituality in social work remains controversial, as it is tainted by the pre-professional era of social work when religion was very much in the forefront. With social work's increasing professionalization, we have attempted to relegate spiritual influences to the background. However, it is clear that the clients of social workers often seek help for problems that involve their religious or spiritual beliefs. And even if it is not immediately obvious, many persons have a spiritual identity that is important to them and should not be ignored or overlooked. In doing an assessment, it is a good idea to be open to spiritual aspects and the role that they may play in the person's adaptation to their world and ability to cope with it. Note that spiritual in the transactional model is not the same as religion; however, it does not exclude the religious. It could be that a better term might be the sublime or the poetic; but spiritual is perhaps more easily understood. We also suppose that the spiritual domain may not always be a factor that guides or drives behavior. In contrast, the biological, psychological, and social domains are prominently evident in human transactions and behavior.

The second caveat is about the number of components. The number of components—biological, psychological, social, spiritual, and challenge in living—could be extended. Some might wish to include the ethical as an additional component for instance, rather than including it under spiritual. The intent of the transactional model is not to limit the perspectives but to capture the diversity of approaches in understanding and helping human beings.

The *challenge in living component* refers to the client's reason for seeking the helping professional or human service agency. The challenge is understood as broader than a presenting problem, and it includes what is known about the challenge and the client's experience of it. It can be understood as a perception of a real-world situation that has biological, psychological, social, and spiritual components. The challenge in living is not necessarily a diagnosis of a physical or mental condition, and it could also be applied to a group of persons. For example, coping with heart disease would be a challenge in living that is experienced by many people. The category of *challenge in living* provides the practitioner with a way to conceptualize something that challenges a person, group, or community, but which is not necessarily a specific mental health term or category.

Such challenge-in-living situations can be conceptualized narrowly or broadly, and the human service professional should use a broad conceptualization to address all the components of the model. This can be illustrated by considering any challenge in living with demographic characteristics such as gender, race, ethnicity, and class. A challenge in living, such as women's problems with substance abuse, could be perceived narrowly as involving only the biological (metabolic differences). Perceived more broadly, such challenges could involve varying degrees of the four aspects: biological, psychological (e.g., rationale for substance abuse among women), social (e.g., loss of appropriate treatment programs for women, especially those who belong to minority cultures or ethnic groups), and spiritual (e.g., effects on spiritual wholeness resulting from the oppression of women over many millennia). In such a broader conception of a challenge, a delimiting demographic would not have an orthogonal location as only one aspect. Rather, it would involve multiple and (as discussed below) simultaneous characteristics and roles in various locations of the model.

Interactions

The transactional model depicts the relationship between the model's five components (see Figure 3.2) in terms of a circular cause-effect-cause perspective, rather than a linear stimulus-response perspective. General systems theory (Seeman, 1989); the ecological model (Germain, 1978); the person-in-environment perspective (Saleebey, 1992); and the concepts of stress, coping,

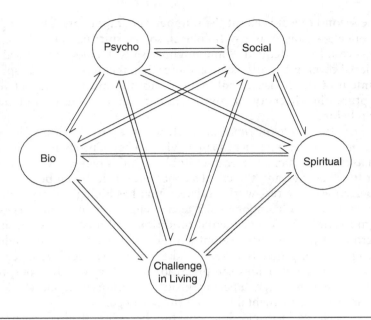

Figure 3.2   Transactional Model for Understanding Neuroscientific Data

and adaptation (Aldwin, 1994) lend theoretical foundations (indicated below) to the model.

The way in which the arrows in Figure 3.2 connect each component (domain) is done to make two main points. First, the simultaneous, interactive interrelationships between the five elements inevitably result in a continual reshifting of the boundaries between the elements. Consider the challenge in living as exemplified by heart disease. As the biological aspects of the illness progress, a person might become psychologically more despondent. This increased despondency may adversely affect significant others in the person's environment (social relationships) so that they also become more pessimistic. The significant others' attitudes may change the psychological boundary by making the patient feel even greater despair. Alternatively, the psychological boundary will shift in the other direction if significant others refuse to feel pessimistic, bolstering the patient with any newly prescribed medicine and making a positive difference in the disease process (spiritual dimension).

Second, moving to a transactional way of thinking from a reductionist or interactionist perspective reflects a paradigmatic change in our way of thinking about health and illness. Aldwin (1994) distinguishes between physiological reductionism, interactionism (where entities interact with each other with no resultant change), and transactionism. Reductionism would show one set of entities being reduced to, or explained in terms of, another. For example, any one or more of the five aspects could be reduced to the physiological or biological aspect. An example of such reductionism is the disease model of illness, which conceptualizes an illness as resulting only from an external agent like a virus or from faulty genes. The transactional model's nonlinearity and dual-direction arrows are intended to rule out this reductionist stance. Interactionism would show several entities interacting and affecting each other but remaining unchanged by the interaction. The paradigmatic shift of the model occurs by drawing attention to the intimate and important involvement of the social, biological, psychological, and spiritual components, especially how they influence each other and evolve as a result. Seeing the domains as evolving as a result of their transactions with each other leads to a truly transactional stance.

Each component of the transactional model is described as a holon, which reflects the idea that each entity or system (i.e., bio-psycho-socio-spiritual challenge in living) is simultaneously a part and a whole (Anderson & Carter, 1984). Each entity faces two directions at once: related inward toward its own parts and outward to the system of which it is a part. For example, looking at the bio system as a holon, we can see that the biological can be a whole entity unto itself. In fact, some with a biological perspective would view human behavior only from this vantage point. But to give the biological system real meaning for use in practice, it should be seen as one part of the total picture. Behavior is not determined by one holon but by the interaction and mutual causation of all the systems and subsystems. So the bio is also part of the psychological, social, and spiritual domains.

Let's consider how we might use the transactional model in our practice. An example of a challenge in living (how the helping professional becomes involved) could be represented by an adolescent male who has recently immigrated to the United States from Central America and is becoming involved in a Latino gang. Rather than seeing his recent emigration as the sole stimulus for his response of getting into trouble via gang membership, the transactional model enables the practitioner to examine the following: (a) the mutual and interacting interrelationships between emigration that affect his sense of self (psychological factor), (b) his intense relations with other gang members from his country of origin (sociocultural factor), (c) the antisocial behavior of gang criminality (possibly a learned behavior), and (d) changing hormone levels in his developing body (biological factor). Each of these factors is unique but contributes to the situation at hand, and each must be addressed by the practitioner, while keeping in mind that all elements are not necessarily equal. For instance, in this example, the effects of emigration on a young boy's developing sense of self (psychological domain) and his very close relationships with other gang members who are from his same country or neighborhood of origin (social factor) are likely to weigh more heavily than the other relevant factors. As we use our understanding of an open system, we can see that all the component parts of this young man's situation are in dynamic interaction with each other. And the resolution or management of this challenge will require attention to these transactions, encouraging the practitioner to search for the varying degrees of biological, psychological, social, and spiritual components in the proposed solution.

Another example is a client who complains of depression and "not being able to accomplish anything." As we gather data about this person in the situation, we find that one's spiritual sense of life and the world has an impact on the depressed mood. Based on this spiritual aspect, the person experiencing depression will respond to social events in a particular way. One's cultural identification may also influence such response. At the same time, the biological aspects of depression (e.g., insufficient amount of serotonin in the brain) could affect the psychological and mental processes such as thinking. These processes might also have an effect on the spiritual life of the person. As a result of looking at the transactions among and between these four variables, we arrive at a more complex—and more helpful—understanding of this person who is experiencing depression. The transactions among the variables will point us in the direction of what needs to be done to improve this person's overall life situation.

Because the transactional model encourages social workers to perceive challenges in living broadly in a context that has bio-psycho-social-spiritual components, one might expect that I am saying that the solution set of problem-solving activities also has the same components. No, the transactional model does not preclude the model user from focusing on particular components of the challenge of living (e.g., on the biological). However, the model does encourage the user to recognize the limits of a single-component approach. It encourages the user to conceptualize the challenges and the solution responses as a simultaneous and interactive series of exchanges. As challenge and solution response mutually affect one another, it suggests an ongoing interactive series or dance.

One more example may demonstrate how the transactional model can be used in clinical practice and how all of the elements of the model do not need to contribute equally to the situation or its resolution. We start with a challenge in living (in this case, an inability to support oneself and to live independently as an adult). This challenge is presented to a case manager who works at a community services board in a medium-size city. After an initial interview, it becomes clear that the 45-year-old male client has been homeless or near-homeless for several months since his mother kicked him out of her home due to his drug use. During the interview, the case manager begins to suspect some kind of mental illness, as the client has great difficulty telling his story and explaining why he is in need of housing, food, and clothing. His vagueness, irritability, and apparent response to voices which the case manager does not hear lead to an initial diagnostic impression of a psychotic disorder. Once previous records are accessed, it is determined that this client has a history with the community services board and has been known by staff there for at least 5 years. How shall the case manager and client dyad proceed?

Refer to Figure 3.2, the *Transactional Model*, which depicts the various domains that need to be addressed to work with this client and help him address his very dire situation. Knowing that this client has a serious and persistent mental illness (probably one of the schizophrenias), the biological domain takes precedence. Based on research findings, the case manager assumes that there is some brain involvement in the client's illness, though the exact brain impairment is unknown. One of the immediate treatment goals would be to assist the client in meeting with a psychiatrist to evaluate the need for psychotropic medication. Again, we know that in some cases, hallucinations and cognitive impairment can be helped by antipsychotic medication. If the client is willing to take prescribed medication, this would have an impact on the other domains. For example, if an antipsychotic was taken, the client's irritability and judgment might be improved, which would enhance his ability to relate to other people and participate in his own treatment. The client's alleged drug use needs to be addressed and can be understood as a biological problem and a social issue. This might entail long-term treatment and include detoxification and/or referral to a Twelve-Step Program. Or perhaps the drug use was a result of lack of treatment for a chronic mental illness, and once the illness is treated, the other substances are not necessary. At this point, it is not known why the client was using street drugs (perhaps to self-medicate his psychotic symptoms; perhaps to fit in with others), but his use created serious problems in the relationship with his mother. Another treatment goal will be to contact the mother to determine what level of social support she (and perhaps other family members) can provide. So the social aspects might be second in the hierarchy of issues to address. Lack of housing and income also need to be addressed immediately (also at the top of the hierarchy) because these are presenting problems; but again, they are intricately related to the biological domain. Until the major mental illness is treated, only bandages can be applied to temporarily fix the housing and income crises.

The psychological domain also comes into play here as we try to assess the role that stress has played in the current situation. Being kicked out of his mother's house would no doubt be quite stressful, and then there is the recent stress of living on the streets and looking for food at homeless shelters and other feeding sites. All of this has contributed to greatly lowered self-esteem. From the initial information gathered by the case manager, there are no data to be placed in the spiritual component. However, this could change at any time and as further information is elicited from this client. By using the transactional model to help us conceptualize this person in his situation, we can see how, when psychotic symptoms are medicated, the client's judgment and his relationship with his mother can improve. Improved judgment makes it more possible for him to accept temporary housing in a shelter and begin the process of applying for Supplemental Security Income based on his disability. So the challenge in living becomes less of a crisis as the biological domain changes and as the social domain is enhanced. If the client's relationship with family members is positively changed as a result of improved mental functioning, the psychological component also is changed. This is of course a very optimistic picture, and in reality, it is quite possible that the client will be unable to follow through with adherence to medications; as a result, he might remain homeless, without funds, and alienated from his mother and family. In this situation, it would seem that the biological is clearly at the top of the hierarchy and is the first component that needs changing, due to the nature of schizophrenia.

Let's now turn to neuroscience and attaching and bonding.

4

Linking to Social Work

Attaching and Bonding

Neuroscience is a valuable link for social work in understanding and facilitating attachment and bonding. It is valuable to the extent that the linking is done within the spirit, as discussed earlier, of the transactional model. The model allows us to consider the bio-psycho-social-spiritual domains of a challenge in living and how they interact with each other and change each other as a result. It is valuable to the extent that we recognize the complexity of the neuroscientific context and the incompleteness of our knowledge. Neuroscientific understandings, especially brain plasticity, can supplement and question attachment theory, which speaks to the relationship of the child and the parent (or another caretaker). The neurosciences can enhance our understanding of human bonding in general.

The "cuddle chemical" is symbolic of the real excitement and the difficulty of neuroscience as it relates to attachment and bonding. The human service professional should share this excitement and use the transactional model as a guide through the difficulties. But he or she should recognize the limitations of such explanations. The cuddle chemical is oxytocin. Oxytocin, like vasopressin, is a hormone that acts as a neurotransmitter within the brain and elsewhere, relaying and modifying electrical signals from neurons to other cells. It has been described in detail, as being a natural hormone, a peptide of nine amino acids, and so on. Oxytocin is released in both genders—during sexual orgasm, for example. It can also be injected into a muscle or a vein. It facilitates birth by causing the uterus to contract, and it helps with breast feeding. More widely, oxytocin is implicated in social recognition and bonding, and it might be an element in forming trust between people.

The "analysis of love has moved from the embrace of poets into the arms of science," declares a Brain Briefing published by the Society for Neuroscience (2006a, p. 1). "Give all to love. Obey thy brain," the Brain Briefing asserts, and "a recent series of precise studies reveals some of the key areas and molecules involved in the ability to love and bond with others" (p. 2). On the contrary, forget shifting from one embrace to another's embrace; no single perspective is enough! The Brain Briefing is enthusiastic, but wrong, to speak about analyses of love going from one set of arms to another single set. Rather, what is required is putting the biological or any other data into the perspective of the transactional model. Despite the biological aspect of oxytocin and vasopressin, which are hormones, isn't love something that is also socially constructed? Isn't love also psychologically constructed and spiritually constructed? As if we need further evidence, isn't the discovery of the plasticity of the brain—to be rediscussed below—incompatible with biological determinism? Human service professionals should not understand biological data passively in a supermarket fashion, as if the data were a display of products among which to search, select, or reject at will. The biological should not be approached on a "show me" basis. Nor should the professional engage in biological triumphalism, thinking that biology has the only arms. Instead, the biological should be engaged, interrogated, and examined in terms of the range of other perspectives—the psychological, social, and spiritual.

Consider first attachment theory, starting with Bowlby's missing link. Then this chapter discusses the more general topic of human bonding.

Attachment Theory: Bowlby's Missing Link

The technological advances of the past 30 years have permitted neuroscience researchers to confirm Bowlby's belief that attachment has a biological link and to highlight what Bowlby did not anticipate: brain plasticity. Through the use of MRI, fMRI, and positron emission tomography (PET) scans, brain structure and function can now be seen in vivo. That is, the structure and functioning can be examined as the subject—human or nonhuman—is awake and performing some task. Two results are especially significant. They point to opportunity for supplementing and transforming attachment theory and for adjusting the conceptualization of the attachment between the child and the parent.

The first result is that neuroscience is John Bowlby's missing link. My point is that neuroscience should be linked to attachment theory. It fits well enough with what Bowlby himself had in mind. Bowlby, a psychoanalyst of the British Object Relations School, first presented his attachment theory in the late 1950s and early 1960s—before the recent neuroscientific revolution. Yet his theory included the idea that attachment is a natural instinctual response that allows for the bonding of infant and mother (Bowlby, 1958, 1959, 1960). Repeat: natural instinctual response!

The second result is the identification of brain plasticity—an even more remarkable finding! The brain alters in response to its experiences, and the way that the brain develops in infancy and early childhood does not necessarily determine the kind of person he or she will become. The concept of brain plasticity enhances—for some, even challenges—attachment theorizing. It bears repeating that early infancy and early childhood do not necessarily determine the persons we will become!

To reflect about the link to attachment theorizing, we consider four items—attachment theory before neuroscience, how neuroscience supports attachment theory (providing Bowlby's missing link), how neuroscience enhances Bowlby's attachment theory (speaking of brain plasticity), and how the theory's foundations should be interrogated (questioned).

Attachment Before Neuroscience

Simply stated, attachment is the emotional connection between an infant and his or her caretaker, especially as it develops over the child's early life. Some use the term *bonding* interchangeably with attachment, and it has been described more specifically as referring to the mother's feelings for her infant (Sadock & Sadock, 2003). Since 1969, when Bowlby reformulated his ideas about attachment, human service professionals have been heavily influenced by attachment theory.

Let's think of attachment theory in terms of three principal theorists: John Bowlby, Mary Ainsworth, and Mary Main.

Bowlby: John Bowlby (1907–1991) used evolutionary theory to explain attachment behavior, which he saw as a guarantee that adults would protect their offspring and ensure their survival. Attachment is thus an expression of a primary and biologically based need for survival of the species. Bowlby referred to the Attachment Behavioral System, which is comprised of the infant and his or her attachment figure—usually the mother—who is relied on as a moderator of anxiety or distress (Bowlby, 1969). In later years, Siegel (1999) described the attachment system as an interpersonal relationship that enables the immature brain of the infant to use the mature brain of the parent to develop its own processes of emotional regulation and social relatedness. This theory seems to echo Bowlby (1951), who described the mother as providing ego and superego functions for her infant during infancy and before the child is able to provide these capacities for him- or herself.

Attachment describes the emotional tone and affective bond between an infant and his or her caretaker(s). Although it develops gradually, by 1 month of age, most infants demonstrate the seeking and clinging behaviors that keep them near the desired person (i.e., the one who will protect them; Sadock & Sadock, 2003). These behaviors become especially strong during age 6 to 12 months and are evident in all cultures (Konner, 2004). In other words, the infant actively engages in relationship development with his or her primary caregiver by building an internal working model, which Bowlby defined as being the infant's internal representations of the self and the other. In Object Relations terms, this working model becomes the template for all future relationships of the infant and developing child. It also can be noted that, based on numerous cross-cultural studies, attachment occurs among nearly all infants, even when the parent is insensitive to and/or mistreats the infant.

Based on what we know of Bowlby's own early experiences, it is appropriate to conclude that someone other than the mother can serve as an attachment figure. According to a recent biography, a nanny and nursemaids provided much of his early care, and his mother and father were much less involved in his raising (Bretherton, 1999). After graduating from the University of Cambridge, he did volunteer work at a school for maladjusted children. This turned out to be a seminal experience that led him to decide on a career as a child psychiatrist. Eventually, he studied at the British Psychoanalytic Institute, which at the time was heavily influenced by Melanie Klein. Although he was supervised by Klein and heavily influenced by Object Relations theory, he disagreed with Klein's approach to the treatment of children. While her treatment of children focused on their fantasies related to conflict between aggressive and libidinal drives, Bowlby, who had studied with two psychoanalytically trained social workers at the London Child Guidance Clinic, believed that what occurred within families was extremely important to the child's emotional disturbance. He believed in the importance of working with parents so that they in turn might help their children, based on his ideas about the intergenerational transmission of attachment relations (Bretherton, 1992). In other words, by assisting parents with their own attachment issues, what they transmit to their children can be modified.

Ainsworth: Mary Ainsworth, a Canadian clinical and developmental psychologist, was a major contributor to the development of attachment theory. She had a lifelong friendship and collaboration with John Bowlby, beginning in 1950. She worked in Bowlby's research unit at the Tavistock Clinic on how separation from mother in early childhood can have an effect on personality development. She greatly extended understandings of attachment theory, including the development of instruments to measure the concept. In 1953, Ainsworth and her husband Leonard moved to Uganda. There, she began an observational study of infants and their mothers among Ugandan villagers. This study, the first empirical study of infant–mother attachment patterns, was later replicated with middle-class families in Baltimore, Maryland. The study results led to the development (in the 1960s) of the Strange Situation attachment classification system.

The Strange Situation was a research procedure that measured 12-month-old infants' reactions to being alone in a room with their mothers, with their mother and a stranger, being alone with the stranger, and then being reunited with the parent. By observing the infant's reactions to these increasingly stressful situations over a period of 20 minutes, Ainsworth and her colleagues assessed the quality and nature of the infant's attachment. As they observed the infant's response to being with his or her mother, left by the mother, and reunited with her, the researchers concluded that there are three categories of attachment. Although 65% of infants were observed to be securely attached, there was also evidence of avoidant and ambivalent attachments (Ainsworth, Blehar, Waters, & Wall, 1978). These types of attachment are also referred to as insecure-resistant (or insecure-avoidant) and insecure-ambivalent. Many studies conducted in different cultures have replicated Ainsworth's findings related to the Strange Situation, and "the majority of infants worldwide have been found secure" (Main, 1996, p. 239). Of the three attachment categories identified, there appears to be more variation among the three categories that exist within a particular country than there is variation between countries. For example, in studies conducted in the United States, maternal sensitivity is reported to be more important for secure attachment in middle-income than in low-income families (Haight, Kagle, & Black, 2003).

Main: The third major contributor to attachment theory was Mary Main, a student of Ainsworth. Building on Ainsworth's Strange Situation, she studied attachment at later ages (e.g., among 6-year-olds). Main and her colleagues found that many infants could not be classified using the Strange Situation. The infants behaved in a conflicted way in the parent's presence, and this led to the identification of an additional type, which she called disorganized attachment style. This category, referred to as Group D, is described as insecure-disorganized-disoriented attachment. Main and Solomon (1990) conclude that approximately 15% to 25% of infants in low-risk samples are considered to be disorganized, based on this fourth category, and the majority of children who are mistreated by their parents also fall into the disorganized attachment category. It is believed that disorganized infants are most at risk for mental disorder, especially dissociative disorders (Main, 1996). What Main does not address is the possibility that children who are identified as having a disorganized attachment style may be experiencing an early onset mental disorder. Another possibility is that these children have suffered early trauma from community violence rather than a lack of parental attachment. As we consider these alternative explanations, we are reminded not to jump to an easy conclusion, when we observe a child who demonstrates insecure-disorganized-disoriented attachment behavior (E. H. Taylor, personal communication, December 3, 2007).

Main also developed the Adult Attachment Interview and found that adult attachment styles correspond to those found in children. In the interview, parents were asked about their own attachment relationships in childhood and how these influenced their development. Based on these 1-hour–long interviews and verbatim transcripts, the researchers identified four main adult attachment classifications, which correspond conceptually and empirically to the infant attachment categories. The adult attachment categories are labeled as secure-autonomous, coherent-collaborative, dismissing, and preoccupied-entangled. One of the more interesting findings of this research is that adults who had unfavorable life histories did not necessarily have insecure offspring. Rather, if they were able to retell their own attachment history in a coherent manner, they were more likely to have secure offspring.

Supporting Attachment: The Link

The neuroscientific link matters! Let's start with the orbitofrontal system of the brain! Neuroscientific research results are enough to confirm that neuroscience is a missing link for the attachment theorizing that Bowlby started. But the association of neuroscientific activity with particular behaviors is not enough to prove a belief that the biological is basic—fundamental, foundational, determinant. Such biological associations are not inconsistent with a claim that, for instance, the cultural is more basic for shaping human behavior, as writers such as Richerson and Boyd (2006) argue—and as I do not. Biological links are consistent with, as another example, the transactional model.

Starting with structure. The biological control system that Bowlby alluded to is now believed to be the orbitofrontal system of the brain (Schore, 2000), a region of the prefrontal cortex (see Figure 4.1). The prefrontal cortex occupies the foremost section of the frontal lobes, which represent a very large portion of the brain and the brain part that distinguishes us humans from other primates. This part of the brain (i.e., the orbitofrontal system) grows substantially during the first 2 years of life, and it has developed enough by the middle of the 2nd year (about age 18 months) that infants have the capacity for a "theory of mind" (Schore, 2003; Wilkinson, 2003). This capacity involves the infant's ability to know how a certain behavior will be perceived by his or her caregiver. Watching a 2-year-old child grabbing a toy away from his younger sister and then looking to his father for a reaction will readily reveal this ability. As a result of the development of this capacity, children are able to adjust their own behavior to get their needs met. This seems to represent the beginning of empathy, and there is some recent evidence that the orbitofrontal limbic system is involved in (mediates) one's ability to empathize (Mega & Cummings, 1994). The orbitofrontal system is also connected to subcortical structures such as the amygdala, through which it receives emotional associations and regulates emotional behavior (Nelson, 2000).

The orbitofrontal system's location, in an area where the cortex (outer layers) and subcortex (underlying areas) meet, allows it to act as a crucial arbiter of cognitive–emotional interactions. It is therefore involved in attachment functions. For example, as the infant sees the face of his or her mother and hears her voice, this information can be joined with emotional processes emanating from

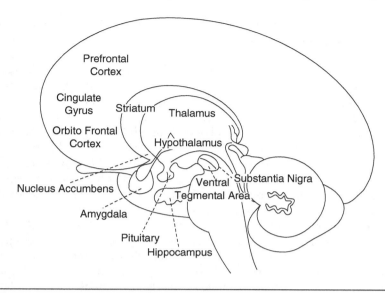

Figure 4.1   Bowlby's Biological Control System (Orbitofrontal System) and Emotional Brain

the limbic system; the orbitofrontal system appraises the cognitive input and assigns emotional meaning. The growth of the orbitofrontal area of the infant's brain occurs especially in the right cerebral hemisphere, that side of the brain that specializes in the processing of social-emotional information and controls the autonomic and endocrinological functions that underlie emotions. The right hemisphere is often seen as more primitive than the left hemisphere, which mediates language, speech, and problem-solving capacities; it is actually more important for what defines a self. For example, the right brain is involved in facial recognition and attention monitoring, which helps to explain human attachment. However, it has been found to be connected to emotional negativity and withdrawal from social relations; and some beginning research demonstrates that one's attachment history may determine how and where certain emotional information is processed (i.e., within the right or left hemisphere; Cohen & Shaver, 2004). The right hemisphere also appears to be involved in the development of psychiatric disturbances, which are often understood as being related to attachment problems or affect dysregulation.

By the end of the 1st year of postnatal life, the child is beginning to stand upright and walk, and the orbitofrontal part of the brain is developing. This is a critical period for the formation of attachment to a primary caregiver, and the infant's capacity for attachment grows out of this period and the affect regulation experiences that have occurred between the infant and the caretaker. During this practicing phase (usually between 10 and 18 months), the infant begins to leave the mother's side and then return. These reunions involve face-to-face and affective communicating. By approximately 18 months of age, the nervous system of the child has been joined symbiotically with the nervous system of the mother, resulting in reciprocal interactions between the regulatory systems of the mother and the infant. Also at this time, there is competition between the sympathetic (energy-expending) and parasympathetic (energy-conserving) limbic structures of the brain, which leads to the maturation of the orbitofrontal system. This entails the child using the mother's sympathetic nervous system to increase his or her arousal level and positive affect (Schore, 1994). Thus, we can see how the maturation of the right hemisphere of the child's brain depends on experiences with his or her caretaker, which in turn leads to the development of brain structures that are able to mediate (serve as a vehicle for bringing about) social and affective functions.

During the 1st year of life, a crucial task for the infant is to develop tolerance for higher and higher levels of arousal. The mother or caretaker enables this by managing and modulating those periods when the infant becomes highly stimulated. As the right orbitofrontal part of the brain develops, the infant becomes better able to tolerate levels of arousal and stimulation. The result is a brain that functions in such a way that it can self-regulate. Conversely, when there is misattunement between the infant and the caretaker, high levels of negative affect result, and this inhibits growth in the very same brain structures (i.e., on the surface and underneath) that regulate affect. Attachment is realized when the positive affect experiences are increased and the negative affect situations are kept to a minimum. Notice that what is important here is not that all affective experiences be positive. Rather, the infant needs to experience more positive than negative.

The neurobiology of these processes is as follows: the right hemisphere of the infant (which processes visual and emotional information such as recognition of mother's face and whether or not the mother's facial expression is stimulating) is psychobiologically attuned to the contents of the mother's right hemisphere (which also is involved with emotional information and nonverbal communication). This very close connection between the infant's and the mother's right hemispheres allows the infant to use the mother's more mature emotion-regulating right hemisphere as the model for imprinting (i.e., attaching to mother) and hard wiring of brain circuits. This connection eventually allows the infant or young child to manage his or her own affective abilities (Schore, 2003).

As we look further into the workings of the right hemisphere, we find much recent research that describes the neural circuitry of this emotional system and how it relates to affective style (Davidson, 1998, 2002). Affective style, which can be described as the quality and intensity of mood and emotional reaction, develops in infancy and in relation to one's primary caretaker. It appears to be related to temperament. Affective style is important, as it helps us to understand why different persons have such different emotional reactions to the same event and why some persons seem to be more vulnerable to psychopathology. Studies have shown that this central circuit of emotion is closely involved with the prefrontal cortex and amygdala, through which cultural aspects, social factors, and genetics are processed (Davidson, 2001; Jackson et al., 2003). Research has also found asymmetries in this neural circuitry, meaning there is a lack of balance between the left and right sides of the brain. For example, greater activation of the left prefrontal cortex is found to be associated with feelings of well-being (Urry et al., 2004).

Continuing with events. In addition to the structural aspects of brain development that are involved in attachment relationships, important biochemical events are also occurring. When the infant sees and is stimulated by the mother's face, large amounts of endogenous opiates are released in the infant's brain, and this explains why the infant feels great pleasure when engaged in this social interaction. As the opiate level increases, dopamine is released, and this leads to further arousal and elation. As the infant continues to gaze at mother's face, levels of corticotrophin releasing factor (CRF) also rise, and this activates the sympathetic part of the autonomic nervous system, which is associated with intense elation, increased arousal, and elevated activity by the infant. Dopamine and endogenous opiates have been found to be in large supply during attachment experiences (as determined by the gaze interaction described above), and the orbito-prefrontal cortex also contains the highest levels of opioids and dopamine found in the cerebral cortex of the brain. The right orbitofrontal area is also involved in storing the memory of emotional faces, based on attachment experiences between mother and infant. The infant develops a schema (i.e., a mental image of mother's face), which is imprinted in the orbitofrontal area of the brain and can be called up in the absence of the mother. This inner representation of mother can be used by the infant to self-regulate emotions.

As the child enters the 2nd year of life, the socio-emotional environment between the caretaker and the child begins to change. What was originally an environment of affection, play, and caregiving must necessarily become more involved with the socialization of the infant. Caretakers begin expressing prohibitions; the child has to learn to restrict exploration and tantrums, and bladder and bowel function become prominent features of daily life. Shame appears around age 14 to 16 months, and this inhibits excitement and joy. The child continues to leave the mother's space and return, but reunions may now involve stress, because the mother's face may have a negative affective quality. The psychobiological processes are also changing. In the presence of stress, corticosteroids are produced, and these reduce the level of opioids and CRF in the brain. The latter is the opposite of what occurred earlier when the infant and the caretaker were beginning to attach. The mother can regulate the shame state by staying with the child who is experiencing this emotion and demonstrating tolerance for the negative affect of her infant. She can then use her face to re-engage with the infant, through smiling. The smile generates positive affect; CRF is released, endorphins are produced, and dopamine flows again.

This process of the infant and parent moving from positive to negative affect and then back again to positive is believed to lead to resilience. Schore (2003) argues that the early relationship between the infant and the mother imprints in the developing right brain of the infant either resilience or vulnerability to future psychiatric disorders (risk or protective factors). If vulnerability is imprinted, the person will be less able to cope with interpersonal stressors for the rest of his or her life.

Structure and events. Indeed, the orbitofrontal system of the right brain plays a critical role in the development of the attachment relationship between the infant and the caretaker; so do events. John Bowlby (1969) argued that the attachment relationship had a direct influence on the infant's ability to cope with stress and that this occurred via the maturation of a biological control system. We now know what Bowlby surmised but could not demonstrate (i.e., this control system is located in the right orbitofrontal system of the brain). Clearly, the neuroscientific link matters!

Enriching Attachment: Plasticity

Brain plasticity is a primary finding from the neurosciences, and it allows for a wider lens for focusing on attachment theory. The idea of plasticity was introduced in 1949 by Donald Hebb (Andreasen, 2001). By learning new information, we can reshape our brains owing to changes at the nerve cell level: thus, there is the saying that "neurons that fire together wire together." In recent years, we have seen a leap forward in recognition of this feature of the brain.

Brain plasticity is exciting to explore, because it renews hope in a person's ability to learn and grow throughout life. Critically, it can be of special significance for clients who have severely intransigent and multiple problems and diagnoses—clients who are crossing our professional paths more frequently and who challenge our competencies. It can give confidence not only to the client but also the client's family members and the client's professional helpers.

What is brain plasticity, what is the evidence, and what is its significance for attachment?

What is plasticity? Plasticity has two elements. The first is that the brain changes throughout life, though this takes place at a much slower rate as we age. Until recently, it was thought that the brain develops and then stops; not so! The changes are lifelong. The brain exhibits an ongoing and large capacity for change. As Restak (2003) puts it, "plasticity refers to the brain's capacity for change. As recently as only a few years ago, most neuroscientists believed that the brain's plasticity largely ceased by adolescence or by early adulthood at the latest. At this point the brain became fixed in its structure and function—at least that was the prevailing assumption" (p. 7). But as Restak indicates, that assumption is wrong.

The second element of plasticity is that the brain alters in response to what it experiences; the brain itself is shaped by experiences. As noted earlier, the way our brains develop in infancy and early childhood does not necessarily determine the kind of person we will become. Again, in Restak's (2003) words, we "now recognize that our brain isn't limited by considerations that are applicable to machines. Thoughts, feelings, and actions, rather than mechanical laws, determine the health of our brain." Importantly, these changes can happen quickly: "For instance, your brain is different today than it was yesterday" (p. 8).

It is now unclear when brain maturation stops and when aging begins. This is a surprising claim that reflects the concept of brain plasticity. What a change from the attitude that maturation ended in, say, adolescence! Sowell, Thompson, and Toga (2004), addressing this question, advise that "long-range serial studies of brain and cognitive changes (accomplishable only in vivo) and combining postmortem and imaging studies" are desirable (p. 390). More information was needed, at the time of their writing, to answer complicated questions about the time line of brain development and aging and the beginning of the brain's decline.

It should be stated that the brain is not completely plastic (e.g., any more than a culture is completely changeable at whim). The character of a brain at one point in time clearly has consequences at a later point in time. Brain functioning can be damaged and, again, partly hard wired. There are limits to plasticity, such as our discussion earlier in this chapter about how the early relationship between the infant and the mother imprints resilience or vulnerability to future psychiatric disorders (Schore, 2003). As a result, a person who reaches age 5 or 6 with certain brain vulnerabilities may be less able to cope with interpersonal stressors in the future, even though his or her brain maintains some plasticity. Genetic endowments (which may also include certain vulnerabilities) and the type and quality-of-life experiences will affect the degree of change that is possible. The negative environments that come from child abuse and neglect have anatomical brain consequences, for example; drug usage is another example. The consequences can include PTSD, depression, and learning problems; and these too will have an effect on the brain. Chapter 3 noted that there are critical periods for the development of the brain (e.g., most of us know that the best time to learn languages is before the teen years). It was also noted in chapter 3 that brain connections follow rules from the genes. Yet the brain is continually changing in response to cultural and other inputs until the moment of death.

Where is the evidence? Through the noninvasive imaging techniques now available (as mentioned earlier) and postmortem inquiries, a mass of literature is now available on brain changes throughout human life—from birth to death. Sowell et al. (2004) summarize this large literature.

It is now established that neurogenesis (i.e., the process by which neurons are created) occurs in the adult brain. Taupin (2005) and Andreasen (2001) are among those researchers who review the supporting literature. This literature began in the 1960s when there was the first evidence that the brain generates new neuronal cells. "Studies in the 1990s confirmed that, contrary to long-held dogma, neurogenesis occurs in the adult brain and that NSCs (neural stem cells) reside in the adult central nervous system" (Taupin, 2005, RA 248). It is thought that neurogenesis originates from neural stem cells. Taupin indicates that the literature highlights "the involvement of adult neurogenesis in a broad range of physiological and pathological processes, widening the function of adult neurogenesis" (RA 250). Although neurogenesis was originally believed to occur only in the hippocampus, where it would be involved in learning and memory, more recently it is thought to occur in other brain areas as well. It has also been found to perhaps play a role (in animal models) in the regulation of stress (Malberg, Eisch, Nestler, & Duman, 2000).

Nancy Andreasen (2001) points to two important components of brain plasticity: critical periods and activity-dependent changes. The idea of critical periods "teaches us that for some aspects of brain development, timing of environmental input is crucial, and that important abilities will be lost or diminished if stimulation does not occur at the right time" (p. 49). The idea of "activity-dependent learning teaches us that exposure to either psychological or biological environmental influences causes changes in the brain" (p. 49). In other words, the kinds of activities and experiences we are exposed to in our environment will determine how our brain changes (i.e., learns; see Figure 4.2).

What is the significance? The significance, I suppose, can be summarized in the claim that we now know that we have a social brain. Eisenberg (1995) puts it well when he speaks of "the social construction of the human brain" (p. 1564).

In thinking about the significance of such plasticity for attachment theory, it is helpful to begin with an image of the newborn human infant and to recall the social nature of brain development. Most of us have had the unique pleasure of seeing and being with a day-old, a week-old, or a month-old infant, either briefly or for extended periods of time. What we observe is a tiny bit of humanity that mainly sleeps, eats, cries, urinates, poops, burps, and seems barely real. But as we watch the new mother, we are likely to see the beginning of an amazing display of relationship. Of course, most mothers, and many fathers, have been working on this relationship for the past 8 or 9 months and already have a sense of who this new little one is and can be. As we know, the fetal brain has also been growing during the in-utero period. At birth, the brain continues to develop in a sequential or hierarchical fashion, meaning that the less complex parts (e.g., the brainstem) develop first and the more complex structures (e.g., limbic system, cortical areas) develop later. It was mentioned in chapter 3 that the brainstem, which

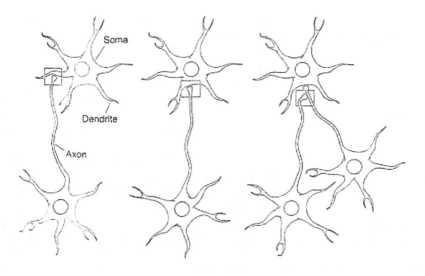

Figure 4.2   Neurons Wiring and Rewiring

regulates cardiovascular and respiratory functions, must be adequately developed at birth for the infant to survive. But the brain's cortical areas, which are involved in cognitive functions, will not mature for many years. The fetal brain and the postnatal brain of the newborn go through a complex process of organization, disorganization, and reorganization. Initially, numerous synaptic connections are made. Following this, excess axons and synapses are eliminated. This is called apoptosis or cell death; it reflects the pruning of synapses (neuronal connections) that were earlier overproduced. This allows for greater complexity in the developing nervous system. Some connections are lost and redistribution occurs based on which connections are most functional for the environment.

It is a reasonable assumption that the attachment relationship between the child and the caregiver during the first 3 years of life is significant for the development of the child's brain. As a result, the environment of the newborn, which is basically a social environment and is managed by the primary caregiver, has an influence on the development of brain structures that underlie the infant's socioemotional development (Schore, 1994). So as we watch a mother "talking" to her infant, smiling (or frowning) with her infant, we notice how she may try to control loud sounds and limit the number of people who come in contact with the newborn. Alternatively, we see that parents are taking their newborn to restaurants and shopping malls within days of being born, and we wonder about how these overwhelming experiences may affect the children. The actions of attuned parents serve to modulate environmental stimulation so that the infant receives enough but not too much. A parent who is in tune with his or her infant will be able to provide this modulation, which eventually is internalized by the infant. This internalization is stored in the infant's memory and can be accessed at a later time. If feelings are not modulated by the parent and the infant is allowed to be overstimulated, the infant internalizes chaos or lack of modulation. This also is internalized and can be called up by the child at a later time.

Our current state of knowledge does not allow us to understand precisely how an impaired right orbitofrontal cortex may lead to difficulties in managing stress. Yet based on observations of social and emotional and bodily functioning, we can begin to understand some behaviors.

Take, for example, a 6-year-old boy in an elementary school setting who demonstrates self-injurious behavior, tantrums, defiance, hyperactivity, short attention span, and impulsivity. Let's call him Warren. Warren is referred to the school social worker because his difficulties with participation in classroom activities are adversely affecting his learning. From the psychosocial history, we learn that this child is the youngest of three children and lives in a two-parent home. Before attending school, this child had little or no contact with children other than his siblings, and his mother reports that he has always been allowed to do whatever he wanted to do and to "have his own way." From this limited information, we can hypothesize that Warren's biological control system (located in the right orbitofrontal cortex of the brain) did not develop appropriately. His relative lack of contact with other children made it impossible for him to read the faces and tones of his peers, and this led to trouble managing feelings between himself and unrelated others. If he was always given his own way, he would not have learned how to cope with early stressors that emerge when children are involved in relationships with each other. Quite possibly, he never had the chance to move away from his mother and toward the unfamiliar. As a result, there was no need to store the memory of mother's face in his orbitofrontal cortex so that it could be called up in his mother's absence. When he went to school and was faced with an array of social and emotional issues, he was unable to retrieve his mother's face, which would serve to help him self-regulate emotions. As a result, 6-year-old Warren is emotionally out of control and unable to successfully manage the school environment. His ability to manage stress is compromised by the gaps in his early social experiences.

Based on traditional thinking, children like Warren will be seen as angry, controlling, and in need of behavioral interventions (consequences) to change his or her behavior. But there is new thinking, based on input from the neurosciences, that understands such children differently. Forbes and Post (2006) believe that parenting of the attachment-challenged child requires something other than behavior modification and consequences, which are usually threatening to the child, fear based, and lacking in empathy. Rather, what is required is that we focus on stress or dysregulation as being the primary culprit and that we help the child to express whatever emotions are behind the stress (usually fear). By so doing, the stress will be calmed, the child will be more able to manage his or her emotions, and behavior will also be more controlled (manageable). So acting out behaviors are understood as being related to stress and fear, which cannot be regulated (managed) by the child.

Social workers should focus on the social brain in approaching attachment theory. Using the transactional model as our guide, we can concentrate on what transpires between the infant and the caretaker (mother) as this relationship develops, with an emphasis on the very early months and years of human development. The infant is a biological being who is intricately related to his or her social environment from the moment of birth. The challenge in living can be understood as the challenge of developing into a fully differentiated adult person. This challenge will be realized to the extent that the biological, psychological, social, and spiritual components of the infant are adequately developed. Each of the dimensions of the transactional model is related to the others, and one dimension can certainly influence another in such a way as to change it. So as the mother or other caretaker talks with the infant and mirrors back certain behaviors, the infant's brain is changed (i.e., the social aspects influence and change the biological). The changed brain in turn will affect the psychological functioning of the infant and the spiritual component. For example, an infant who receives mirroring input from his or her caretaker will develop more synaptic connections in the areas of the brain that are developing. In using attachment theory, social workers and other human service professionals can benefit by remembering about the social construction of the brain.

Foundations of Attachment?

Social workers should re-examine the foundations of their attachment (pardon the pun!) to attachment theory. For the past 35 years, the importance of attachment theory has been generally accepted among those who are interested in and who provide services to children and parents, and there is a tendency in disciplines to stick with the same questions and with existing theoretical constructs. Most disciplines incline to regard traditional approaches as the dictates of common sense. So it seems commonsensical to view the attachment that develops between an infant and its primary caretaker as the most important predictor of how the child will develop and the prime determinant of the psychological health of the adult. Two questions arise, however. Is attachment theory designed, unconsciously perhaps, with a sociopolitical objective? Is attachment between child and parent transferable, even in later life, to other kinds of human bonding?

Consideration of these questions underscores the desirability for social workers to reflect on their disciplinary and personal preferences.

Political. Some see the focus on attachment as having more political than clinical relevance (Kagan, 1992). In an era when most mothers of young children are employed outside the home and must use day care arrangements for their children, society can be viewed as supporting the idea of attachment as a way of promoting the important bond between the parent and the child. It does seem that we are loath to discuss such issues; and perhaps we readily accept the idea of attachment without critical appraisal of it. Perhaps the concept of attachment has been socially constructed in accordance with a political objective. It is clear enough that the concept is not a biological reality, independent of how we think. Perhaps the concept is sociopolitical.

The author of *The developing mind: Toward a neurobiology of interpersonal experience*, child psychiatrist Daniel Siegel, was astonished to be invited to visit with Pope John Paul II. According to the e-mail that invited him, the pope wanted to know why "the mother's gaze" was so "critical to the growth and emotional well-being of a baby" (Wylie, 2004, p. 29). Recall the devotion to Mary, Jesus' mother! Wylie tells us that Siegel wanted the pope to know ahead of the visit that the gaze could come from either parent or from another attachment figure. If not the pope, then many others do attach importance to such features of attachment theory—for their own sociopolitical principles.

The focus on the mother is a charge that some feminist writers also bring against attachment theory. Susan Contratto (2002) argues that attachment theory can be put to profoundly conservative uses. Diane Eyer (1990) also claims that study of postpartum mother-infant bonding shows that research programs conducted in the 1970s were poorly constructed because they were politically useful in the "struggle between advocates of natural childbirth and managers of the medical model of birth" (p. 71). Her study analyzes "the processes by which one body of scientific research was transformed into a myth. It is a story in which there are no true villains except delusion, no true heroines except the zeal to reform" (p. 69). She characterizes the "discovery" as "rooted in the institutional needs of medicine and in popular beliefs about the true nature of motherhood" (p. 84). Susan Franzblau (1999), on parallel lines, contends that the ideology of control applied to women's reproductive capabilities is implicitly structured in the language of attachment. Language in this case can be interpreted in narrower and broader senses, and I think that it helps to frame such claims if the broader sense is used. In the narrower sense, language consists of items such as grammar and syntax. In the broader sense, language is a matter of cultural perspective. The former is items like grammar and syntax; the latter is a matter of cultural perspective. The unconscious urge to control women is, in this view, part of the unconscious language of attachment.

The issue of the political in attachment theory need not be an either-or matter. For instance, there could be a mixture of motivations and attitudes, both conscious and unconscious. What comes to mind is a form of the talking cure; social workers and other clinical practitioners should talk about such possible foundations of attachment theory.

Transferable? Is the extent of success of early attachment between child and parent transferable to other relationships (e.g., to the various kinds of more general human bonding)? Not everyone believes so.

Some argue that the attachment hypothesis (i.e., that the nature of the mother–infant bond during the early years of life will determine the kind of adult the child becomes) should not be considered as an absolute principle (Kagan, 1997; Tronick, 2003). Although Kagan does not discount the importance of the primary relationship between the infant and the mother, he believes that it is inaccurate to think that a specific early attachment relationship will inevitably result in a specific group of consequences for later relationships. He thinks that it is foolish to try to apply such an equation to all children. Tronick believes that the original mother–infant relationship is unique and develops a "thickness," which is not transferable to other or later relationships. This makes future relationships uniquely different from the original. As a result, the original relationship does not serve as a prototype for all future relationships.

Let's consider Jerome Kagan's (1997) view in more detail. He criticizes the belief that out of the primary attachment relationship there develops a certain type of early experience that continues to remain stable over time. The intervening variable (for Kagan) between parenting behaviors and child outcomes is temperament. So what do we mean when we refer to a child's or an adult's temperament? It generally refers to a quality that is inherited, but it is not considered to be a personality type. It describes something that a child is born with, a potential that is acted on by environment. Therefore, temperament is not totally biological but represents collaboration between biology and experience. It is derived from one's physiology, but environmental events such as climate and diet also influence one's temperament. We might hear someone refer to another person as being temperamental. This usually has the connotation of being difficult. It is in this sense that the word can be described as an emotional bias. The emotional component is stressed, and it consists of one's susceptibility to certain emotional states, the intensity of a specific state, and one's ability to regulate such states (Kagan & Snidman, 2004).

The idea of temperament has been with us for a very long time. Ancient Greeks and Romans described different types of persons based on the four humors: yellow bile, black bile, blood, and phlegm. The four humors were present in all people, but the varying amounts of each would determine the type of person that resulted. I suppose that the word *temperament* was chosen to reflect the mixture of humors: The word is derived from the Latin word *temperare*, meaning to mix. In the 2nd century AD, the physician Galen described nine temperamental types that originated from the four humors. Based on his idea of the dominant qualities, Galen coined four temperamental categories: melancholic, sanguine, choleric, and phlegmatic.

The idea of infant temperament was reintroduced in the late 1950s by Thomas, Chess, and Birch (1968), psychiatrists who studied infants by interviewing their parents. From this research, they developed nine temperamental dimensions and eventually three categories of temperament: the easy child, the slow-to-warm-up child, and the difficult child. In more recent years, Kagan and his colleagues (Herschkowitz, Kagan, & Zilles, 1997; Kagan & Snidman, 2004) have continued to study infant and child temperament, but with a focus on brain measures, emotions, and behaviors of children when they are confronted with the unfamiliar. They have focused on two types of temperament (though it is understood that there exists a large variety of temperaments). The two types are inhibited and uninhibited, and they are somewhat akin to Carl Jung's introverted and extroverted personality types. Inhibited temperament refers to a child who responds to the unfamiliar with wariness and avoidance and can be described as shy or timid. This type is also referred to as high-reactive, in the sense of being temperamentally biased toward high reactivity in the presence of the unknown. Uninhibited temperament refers to a child who is sociable and bold and approaches the unfamiliar stranger eagerly. This type is referred to as low-reactive when confronted with an unknown stranger or situation.

Infants, children, and adolescents from both of Kagan's (1994) temperamental categories—inhibited and uninhibited—have been studied extensively, including assessments on biological variables and their relation to behavior. Some of the biological variables studied include heart rate, blood pressure, pupillary dilation, muscle tension, cortisol levels in saliva, electroencephalographic asymmetry, brain stem auditory-evoked response, and levels of neurotransmitters such as dopamine, serotonin, and norepinephrine. It is now believed, though not proven, that high and low reactive properties are physiologically based in the neurobiology of the amygdala (Kagan & Snidman, 2004), which is a small, almond-shaped organ that lies deep within the brain. The amygdala influences—as discussed later—one's reaction to novelty and instructs the body to flee, freeze, or fight. It acts like a central command post for sensory information and mediates emotions and actions. Based on this hypothesis, high-reactive persons (inhibited temperament) seem to have a more excitable amygdala and also demonstrate higher values on some of the biological variables (e.g., more reactive sympathetic nervous system, higher level of muscle tension, and greater cortical arousal to new experiences). These are the people who generally have a dislike for excessive novelty and are more likely to have social phobia. Low-reactive persons (uninhibited temperament) have a less excitable amygdala and lower values on biological variables; these people are attracted to new experiences.

The question remains of how an infant's temperament might affect the attachment relationship. It seems to me that the infant's temperament interacts with that of the parent or caretaker and influences how the parent or caretaker will respond. Evidence for this mechanism can be seen in families with more than one child, where the same parents develop attachment relationships of a different quality with each child. At a minimum, however, Kagan (1992) can be interpreted as warning that structure and functioning of the brain are not fixed by the parent–child outcome. For Kagan, one's temperament can change, and therefore, an adult is not destined to maintain specific qualities that were predicted from childhood.

Bonding (and Oxytocin)

Oxytocin is reoffered as a symbol of the importance of the neurobiological for social work understanding of human bonding. Yet the social worker must cut through the rhetorical and contested claims that make understanding difficult. In interpreting and appreciating the evidence for the role of brain chemicals such as oxytocin, we need to recognize the complexities of neurobiological structure and functioning. Considering this complexity, one must also appreciate that neurobiological explanations often reveal only parts of the picture; the veil is not lifted in a single flourish. We must expect tentativeness and even conflicting interpretations of the complete picture (e.g., tentativeness in understanding the meanings of terms such as bonding, conflicting interpretations about the relevance of animal studies for understanding of human bonding). For complex and multiple systems, simple answers are rarely simply available.

Interpretation

It needs to be recognized that oxytocin plays a significant role in the bonding process. In other words, what is oxytocin a neural signature of? (A neural signature is the neural representation of something like a behavior or a concept). Neural signatures should be a concern for social workers when considering oxytocin and bonding.

What bonding role? Human bonding concerns relationships not only between the caretaker and the child but also between other humans. Such bonds range from pairs (as in a child–parent or other couple relationships) to groups (as in family relationships or societal bonds); that which keeps societies as collective and functioning entities. Within this range, there is variety. In his attachment theory, for example, John Bowlby (1958) spoke of the affectional or emotional bond. John Money (1986), as another example, writes about the erotic bond.

Beyond the human, there is also human–animal bonding, as some of us feel for our pets. Like most social workers, I want to evaluate the role of oxytocin in terms of human bonding.

Role in love? I agree with Sue Carter (2004) in her essay on "Oxytocin and the Prairie Vole"; love is also open to a wide range of interpretations. The neurobiology of love encompasses a variety of different definitions, ranging from compassion (e.g., reacting to the death of a loved one) to passion (e.g., falling in love) and beyond (e.g., holding a newborn baby). Included in most definitions is an idea of human bonding, even though that, too, is socially constructed. But her claim is not that the bonding is biologically determined. Carter describes such bonds as more likely to be formed during periods of vulnerability. Her examples include birth, lactation and nursing, sexual interactions, and periods of distress. Although she does not express it in these terms, this view treats the child–mother relationship described by Bowlby (1958) as a special case of a more general understanding of the biological and other features that encourage bonding.

Bonding has other roles and relevance. Difficulties in human bonding have medical implications, for example, that are important for social workers helping ill persons and their relatives, in hospitals and other settings. As Carter (2004) points out, social bonds can increase survival chances: "in humans a sense of social support is associated with a more successful recovery from cardiovascular disease, cancer, and mental illness and reduces the vulnerability to substance abuse" (p. 55). She adds that more than one study shows that predictors of vulnerability to many diseases are indices of social support (e.g., Uchino, Cacioppo, & Kiecolt-Glaser, 1996). Such bonds are also important in terms of adapting to changes in environment. This is familiar, in different terminology, to social workers who conduct support groups to help victims of particular illnesses, such as support groups for cancer survivors, or for persons with mental illness. It is also the reason why we so ardently try to involve family and/or significant others in a person's life when he or she is in a vulnerable or problematic situation. We may not think explicitly of such social support examples as human-bonding agencies, but they are.

Here, we limit ourselves to human affectional bonding in general terms.

Neural signatures. Social neuroscience includes assessing the neural signature of a human behavior such as bonding, just as it includes the tracking of other mental states. Deconstruction of concepts and their meaning is described by Decety and Keenan (2006) as a concern of social neuroscience.

Decety and Keenan (2006) explain that many of the existing concepts that social neuroscientists encounter need to be deconstructed because they do not map directly onto neural processes (i.e., what goes on in the brain). Surely, it would merit reflection (and adjustment) if I have one concept for process X (e.g., bonding) and more than one neurological process for X. I am interested if I have any mismatch between concepts and neural processes (e.g., two concepts and one neural arrangement, etc.). Decety and Keenan give the examples of moral dilemma, empathy, and self-regulation—items that relate to human bonding. In these cases, there are disconnects between the way we think and neurological facts. D. J. Farmer (2007) gives a different example to explain what deconstruction means in this context. The example is thinking about loving. If we want to think with clarity about loving, it is helpful to deconstruct the place of the heart in loving. Regarding the function of the heart, we still tend to think under the influence of a misunderstanding held by those such as Aristotle. Aristotle considered the heart to be the center of the intellect. It is antiquated and misleading to declare "I love you with all my heart," and it can mislead even distinguished thinkers—as when Blaise Pascal (1670/1995), French mathematician, philosopher, and physicist, made his famous claim that "the heart has its reasons which reason knows nothing of." The point here is not to oppose the writing of Valentine cards or to encourage people to declare "I love you with all my pump"; it is to give an example of a disconnect, open to deconstruction, between modern thinking and modern biology. This can be explained more clearly by considering human bonding in terms of evolutionary psychology, which combines cognitive psychology and evolutionary biology (Evans & Zarate, 1999; Pinker, 1997). Evolutionary biology regards the brain and mind as operating with modules that have a specific purpose. That is, the brain is not a general purpose processer. These modules, having evolved by natural selection, are designed to solve a particular adaptive problem in a particular context. Examples are the problems of avoiding predators, eating the right food, forming alliances, helping children and other family members, reading other people's minds, and selecting mates.

Second, another leading view is that these mind modules were developed 100,000 or more years ago when the context was different (e.g., group size was smaller)—on the African savannah, where our adapting ancestors lived. These modules implicate multiple neural pathways (see the two neural pathways for fear alarms, discussed below). Identifying neural signatures is common in animal studies (e.g., identifying the neural signature of taste familiarity in the gustatory cortex of the freely behaving rat; Bahar, Dudai, & Ahissar, 2004), which is important to rats wanting to eat unpoisoned food. Identifying neural signatures includes human studies, some related and some unrelated to bonding issues. Related to human bonding are studies like that searching for a neural signature of self-consciousness, discussed in chapter 2. Social workers need to pay attention to social neuroscience as it unravels the various neural signatures of bonding, so that we can have a fuller understanding of human bonding and its protective factors throughout the life cycle.

Rhetoric

How are language and images used to influence and persuade people by other than rational means? On the topic of bonding, naive and simple reporting is common. "There is a tendency in public journals to report oversimplistic interpretations of complex issues," comments Decety and Keenan (2006, p. 6). But the problem is not limited to rhetoric. Inevitably within any science, there are disagreements in interpretations, and often the results are later challenged.

The rhetoric (i.e., language) of neuroscience and human bonding, like most rhetoric, is a mixture of some fantasy, some hopeful news, and some bad news—and, of course, some truth. Here are six examples:

- Let's invent an Oxytocin Meter, declares a *New York Times* Op-Ed piece called "Of human bonding." "Oxytocin is a hormone that helps mammals bond" (Brooks, 2005, p. 11, col. 1).
- A love hormone! "A nasal spray containing a 'love hormone' may actually help defuse marital squabbles, scientists reported" (Reinberg, 2006, p. 1), commenting on the proceedings of the International Congress of Neuroendocrinology in Pittsburgh.
- Reuters News Service (2006) reports that "intranasal administration of oxytocin causes a substantial increase in trusting behavior." It also added some bad news, offsetting the good news—it "could be a criminal's dream drug—a hormone that makes people trust you."
- The British Broadcasting Corporation (2006) reports more bad news, noting Antonio Damasio's worry that "political operators will generously spray the crowd with oxytocin at rallies of their candidates."
- "Trust potion of oxytocin not just fiction anymore," declares the WebMD (2006), "A whiff of oxytocin (has been) shown to increase trust . . . (T)he news comes from scientists, not the Brothers Grimm."
- Here's some more news, both good (from a financial advisor's perspective) and bad (from an investor's perspective), in an article titled "Oxytocin—don't sniff if you want to hang on to your money!" "A new study has concluded that sniffing a substance that occurs naturally in everyone's body makes people trust others with their money" (Medical Studies/Trials, 2006).

Contested Claims

The problem of contested claiming—and the associated uncertainty—is not limited to the press, however. Scientific interpretations are often involved in contested claiming. This is the case with oxytocin, which is related to human bonding; but it is also claimed that people's bonding and other behavior is governed by the "selfish gene" (Dawkins, 1976), mentioned in chapter 2.

There are also other areas that provide examples of contested claiming. Recall the excitement about the "smart gene" or the "IQ gene"—with its possibilities for our children. In 1999, it was claimed that the ability of mice to learn a maze was enhanced by inserting a gene associated with memory. Routtenberg, Cantallops, Zaffuto, Serrano, and Namgung (2000) put it, "Here we show that genetic overexpression of the growth associated protein GAP-43, the axonal protein kinase C substrate dramatically enhanced learning and long-term potentiation in transgenic mice" (p. 7657). As a news report put it, scientists "have engineered mice that, in mazes, can run rings around ordinary rodents"

(Whitehouse, 2000, p. 1). On the Human Genome Project Web site, the U.S. Department of Energy (n.d.) comments, "Once news of the 'smart gene' reaches the public, suddenly there is talk about designer babies and the potential of genetically engineering embryos to have intelligence and other desirable traits, when in reality the path from genes to proteins to development of a particular trait is still a mystery."

Claims at the cutting edge, like that about oxytocin, inevitably involve some uncertainty—unknowns, imperfectly knowns, and not-yet knowns. On the same lines as erotic bonding, we can read in the third edition of a standard neuroscience textbook that the "more complex aspects of sexual behavior and the brain systems that generate them are still quite mysterious" (Bear et al., 2007, p. 561).

Sorting through the rhetoric—the good news, the bad news, and the truth—and contested claims requires practical and critical judgment from the human service professional and ongoing attention to social neuroscience. It also requires understanding of the nature of scientific activity, especially some understanding of philosophy of science. It's a sorting that requires attention both to the missing link and to the transactional model.

Evidence for Oxytocin's Role

There are the prairie vole and other animal studies. These studies suggest that bonding in these animals implicates oxytocin and vasopressin, acting through brain areas that produce rewarding feelings of pleasure. Let there be no misunderstanding, however. There is a veritable cottage industry of such studies, and the number is increasing over time (e.g., as evidenced by the number of reports at recent annual conferences of the Society for Neuroscience).

What a research opportunity! Prairie voles are mouse-like rodents, living in the American Midwest. They are models—poster voles, as it were—for monogamy. The male and the female form a tight pair bond and live in the same nest. They work together in rearing their offspring, and the male defends his mate with determination. Then there are the prairie vole's cousins, the meadow voles. Although very similar genetically and in other ways, the meadow voles have an utterly different mating and living strategy. They are promiscuous. The male and female live in separate nests. The male takes no part in parenting, and the meadow vole mother does so only briefly. But there are differences between the two kinds of vole in terms of receptors for oxytocin and vasopressin.

Oxytocin and vasopressin have been found to be involved in social bond formation in prairie voles. In prairie voles, which are monogamous, there are more receptors for oxytocin (in females) and for vasopressin (in males) in brain areas of the mesolimbic dopamine pathway and opioid systems; the latter are brain circuits involved in reward (Insel, 1997; Young, Lim, Gingrich, & Insel, 2001). Young and Wang (2004) report that differential regulation of oxytocin and vasopressin receptors can explain differences between species' abilities to create pair bonds. Lim, Murphy, and Young (2004) also report on the crucial roles played by oxytocin and vasopressin receptors in the establishment of pair bonds in our friend, the monogamous prairie vole; so does another study by Lim et al. (2004). Earlier, Cho, DeVries, Williams, and Carter (1999) found that pretreatment with oxytocin and arginine vasopressin increases the preference of prairie voles to cohabit with a single mate; it affects preference formation. In the more promiscuous meadow vole, there is less vasopressin in the forebrain. To simplify, changing the quantity of vasopressin reduces the promiscuity. Furthermore, during the brief time when she does parent her offspring, the promiscuous meadow vole registers an increase in her oxytocin.

In another study where researchers observed mother rats and their offspring shortly after birth, it was found that mothers who engage in greater amounts of licking and grooming (LG, as it is called) of their pups (i.e., high LG mothers) have offspring who as adults are less fearful and show more modest hypothalamic-pituitary-adrenal axis responses to stress than do pups who are raised by low licking and grooming (low LG) mothers (Liu et al., 2001). What seems to contribute to the high LG behavior is that high LG mothers have increased estrogen sensitivity that enhances oxytocin activity, and this in turn increases dopamine release. But when high LG mothers are exposed to stress, they become low LG mothers. The researchers conclude that stress appears to diminish parental investment in their young, which in turn results in the offspring being more reactive to stress. The biological mechanism of action in these instances appears to be that maternal care very early in the life of the rat may program the expression of certain genes in the brain, therefore having an ongoing effect in the life of the animal. But there is an additional interaction between gene and environment. In the example above, the offspring of low LG mothers experienced greater amounts of stress reactivity, which may be adaptive for the environment that they inhabit. Although these studies were conducted on rats, Meaney (2004) argues that similar effects occur in humans.

This research focuses on nonhuman animals, of course, but if these two neuropeptides—oxytocin and vasopressin—are crucial for affiliative behavior and social attachment in prairie voles and similar animals, perhaps they also function similarly in humans. Much of the basic neuroscience research is conducted on laboratory animals such as rats because there are fewer ethical restraints and there are substantial commonalities between the brains of all vertebrate species.

On one hand, Bartels and Zeki (2004) tell us that "almost nothing" is known about the corresponding neural correlates in the human brain. On the other hand, the more basic the research is, the more likely it is to be relevant, even when there appears to be a distant relationship of the subject to humans. There is evidence from primates—our closest relatives—that oxytocin facilitates nurturing behavior in females and sexual aggressiveness in some males. There is also some suggestive research on humans. The Bartels and Zeki (2004) study just mentioned, for instance, includes a report that maternal love and romantic love involve brain regions rich in oxytocin and vasopressin brain receptors. As another example, there is the study of 18 children who were raised in Russian or Romanian orphanages as infants and then adopted by American families. Several years after being adopted, they were compared with a group of 21 children who were raised by biological parents in a healthy home environment (Fries, Ziegler, Kurian, Jacoris, & Pollak, 2005). All children participated in interactive computer games in the company of their mother or another woman. Following the task, a urine sample was taken and oxytocin and vasopressin levels were measured. Results showed that the children who had spent their early years in neglectful environments (the orphanages) did not demonstrate an increase in oxytocin level following physical interaction with their mothers, whereas the control group children did demonstrate an oxytocin jump. Children in the experimental group also produced lower levels of vasopressin, a hormone that is important for recognizing a person as being familiar. This recognition ability is seen as being necessary for forming social bonds. Yet another example is a report that oxytocin and vasopressin receptors are activated when mothers look at photographs of their own children but not when looking at photographs of other people's children. It was mentioned earlier that oxytocin is involved in human social behaviors (e.g., milk release during nursing). In these and other ways, the animal results are being applied in human studies—and are now being researched in social neuroscience.

Bruce Wexler (2006, pp. 86-88) highlights three features of oxytocin, emphasizing that it is a "social neuropeptide unique to mammals." First, oxytocin plays a role, as I have indicated, in maternal behaviors. Second, it is significant in social behavior more broadly. For instance, "When the gene that directs the synthesis of oxytocin is knocked out, and the mice are unable to make oxytocin, they are completely unable to recognize other mice, even after repeated encounters with them" (p. 87). Third, as just indicated, oxytocin is found only in mammals: "It is thus a concrete marker of the defining importance of social interaction in the development and life of mammals" (p. 88).

Complexities

Both biological and nonbiological features in interaction complicate any evaluation of the role of oxytocin. Here, I focus on the biological. But societal features and actions, clearly significant, add no less to the complexities of understanding human bonding (e.g., war, peace, the power plant disaster in Chernobyl, September 11, etc.).

The biological complexities result from features such as the nature of individual neuroscientific processes, the multiplicity of relevant processes, and the ongoing character of the neuroscientific revolution. Individual neuroscientific processes are nothing if not complex: Some specialists like to say that the human brain is the most complex entity in the universe. Examples abound from almost any aspect of neuroscience (e.g., the array of neurotransmitters, the variety of receptors, and the multitude of ion channels involved in some synaptic transmissions). Take signaling with a single neuron, for instance; this can be described as resembling "in some ways the signaling of the neural networks of the brain itself" (Bear et al., 2007, p. 164).

The multiplicity of relevant processes for human bonding can be illustrated by recalling behavior connected with levels of serotonin, unrelated to oxytocin. (In this example, recall that level of aggression is related to human bonding.) An inverse relationship has been shown between levels of serotonin and aggression (or antisocial attitudes and behavior). In an essay on social neuroscience, Suomi (2004) describes his work on rhesus monkeys. He points out that the capability for aggression is desirable among monkeys for survival in the wild. Yet the rough-and-tumble aggression that the monkeys exhibit at the age of 6 or so months of age must be socialized. Suomi describes his work in establishing a link between violent and antisocial aggressive behaviors and "deficits in serotonergic functioning, as indexed by unusually low concentrations of the primary central serotonin metabolite 5-hydroxyindoleacetic acid (5-HIAA) in the monkey's cerebrospinal fluid" (p. 18). To give a different example, the multiplicity of relevant processes is pointed out, for love, when Carter (2004) again points to the importance of the chemistry of reward to processes that permit attachments: "Central to the theories of reward is the catecholamine dopamine" (p. 58). The study, noted above, by Cho et al. (1999) implicates dopamine-oxytocin interactions in their prairie vole study. Carter also points out that the chemistry of love shares common elements with addiction (e.g., reliance on dopamine).

The multiplicity of relevant responses for human bonding can also be illustrated by considering the neurological features of emotional responses—clearly related to bonding. Behavior is shaped by parts of what some have called the "emotional brain"—mainly the amygdala, the hippocampus, the anterior cingulate cortex, and the hypothalamus. It was mentioned earlier that LeDoux (1996) describes the behavior response to fear alarm in terms of a low and a high road. He describes two neural pathways. The amygdala works on the low road; the high road is through the prefrontal cortex. One pathway through the amygdala results in the body freezing with fear at the sight of the potential danger. Another pathway leads milliseconds later to the awareness that the situation is really not dangerous; and when the person decides that the situation is really not dangerous, he or she can then unfreeze.

Let's clarify by describing this complex dual process in more detail. The amygdala receives and interprets stimuli and specifies action (e.g., fight or flight, eat or abstain). Its main involvement is with stimuli that implicate fear, danger, threat, or embarrassment, but it also interprets stimuli associated with highly emotional features such as envy, disgust, frustration, affection, and love. One important point is that the amygdala learns and remembers what to fear (i.e., there is conditioned fear and response, the Pavlovian reflex that can associate the sound of a bell and the teeth of a savage dog). The amygdala does this in addition to processing information about complex social states, intentions, and relationships (see Adolphs, 2006). Another point is the readiness of unconscious responses—except in those with autism—to human facial expressions (e.g., to fear and aggression in such expressions). The amygdala, on the low road, handles situations on a quick and dirty basis (e.g., the car is approaching quickly, I'm in the middle of the road, and I have to jump now). If my amygdala were damaged, there would be no such response. The hippocampus influences the amygdala and the hypothalamus to regulate the reactions of the autonomic nervous system. It is involved with context-dependent memories—the declarative memory, mentioned in chapter 2. It recognizes facts and remembers the context of the facts. The hippocampus, like the amygdala, is involved in memory formation. The hippocampus is involved with nonemotional memories, whereas the amygdala is concerned when the memory formation is highly emotional. The anterior cingulate cortex limits the amygdala to temper negative emotions, providing for conflict resolution and human socialization. It is involved in problem solving and emotional self-control. Detecting conflicts between plans and action, it acts on the prefrontal cortex—especially the orbitofrontal cortex—and the insula to serve a warning. It contains neurons concerned with ameliorating distress. The hypothalamus influences the emotions by acting like a thermostat and thereby controlling homeostasis. It operates through the autonomic nervous system (e.g., blood pressure, temperature, hormone secretion, and energy).

The multiplicity of relevant responses for human bonding can be illustrated by many other examples. One such example is the functioning of social chemosignals (e.g., pheromones). As Martha McClintock (2004) explains, these chemosignals can allow social interactions to regulate neural and endocrinal events. She notes that women produce pheromones when ovarian follicles are ripening, and these "accelerate ovulation in other women and shorten their menstrual cycles. In contrast, when women ovulate, their pheromones have the opposite effect on other women, delaying their ovulation and lengthening their menstrual cycles" (p. 65).

The neurobiological complexity of constructing my sense of self and other is another example of the multiplicity of responses relevant for human bonding. On the sense of self, the neurological component—even though not determinative—is surely an unconscious contributing factor to my sense of self. For instance, it contributes to my image of my body (e.g., Goldenberg, 2005). As Restak (2006) reports, "As illustrated by Ehrsson's (rubber hand) experiment, the boundaries and qualities of our sense of self are a good deal more malleable than we might predict" (p. 93). On the construction of the self, Patricia Churchland (2002) reminds us that "The key to figuring out how a brain builds representations of 'me' lies in the fact that, first and foremost, animals are in the moving business; they feed, flee, fight, and reproduce by moving their body parts in accord with bodily needs. This modus vivendi is strikingly different from plants, which take life as it comes" (p. 70). On the other hand, there is the matter of whether the "other" is constructed in my mind as someone worthy of empathy or someone worthy only of the back of my hand. As Restak (2006) points out, "Empathy involves a similar blurring of the boundary between self and other" (p. 93). Later in his chapter on "The empathic brain: Blurring the boundaries between self and others," he notes that "empathy involves sensitivity not only to the other person's experience but to our own as well. We can feel another's pain only if at some earlier point in our life we've experienced pain ourselves" (p. 93).

The ongoing character of the neuroscientific revolution reflects the fact, that despite the quantum achievements of recent decades, much remains to be discovered and much is imperfectly known. Recall Bear et al. (2007), quoted earlier, about the lack of understanding regarding aspects of sexual behavior and the brain systems that generate them. Carter (2004) says that, even though the "experience of love and the causes and effects of social bonds are based on ancient neural and endocrine systems . . . the exact chemistry of human love remains to be described" (p. 61); the relevant research is in its infancy.

So we should be neither surprised nor discouraged when returning to the Society for Neuroscience's (2006a) Brain Briefing about oxytocin, noted earlier. It comments on the relevance of the studies on the prairie voles: "Although it's still not clear how the findings translate to humans, some research indicates that these hormone systems may malfunction in people who have difficulties with social interaction." Furthermore, "More work is needed to clearly decipher the brain's involvement in love and bonding. Regardless, much evidence already says that many valentines, ballads, and romantic poems warrant a revision, at least for accuracy's sake." Oxytocin and vasopressin matter.

Understanding?

The neuroscientific revolution challenges human service professionals to rethink about attaching and bonding, both the foundations and the content. Attachment theory is enhanced by what we have called Bowlby's "missing link" and by the discovery of the plasticity of the brain. Its foundations can be questioned in such terms as political motivation and transferability. As a result, the theory is opened up. It deserves reiteration that attachment theory should be seen in the context of human bonding.

Human bonding is also enhanced and challenged by its link to neuroscience. Oxytocin is taken as symbolic of the challenge—a symbol that could as well have been the humble prairie vole. The claim is that there are neurobiological factors that encourage human bonding, and social workers should recognize them. But the claim is not that the bonding is biologically determined. Sue Carter's (2004) claim was that such bonds are more likely to be formed during periods of vulnerability. This view treats the child-caretaker relationship described by Bowlby as a special case of a more general understanding of the biological and other features that encourage bonding.

It has been proposed that social workers should seek to understand these neurobiological factors by moving toward social neuroscience. The issue is not confined to what social workers can get off the shelf from social neuroscience. Recall the admonitions earlier in this chapter to the effect that the social worker should not understand biological data passively in a supermarket fashion and that the biological should not be approached on a "show me" basis. I want to reemphasize what social workers can bring to the social neuroscience table. We come again to the transactional model.

Such is the fecundity of neuroscience that pursuing the topic of human bonding in the social neuroscientific setting will produce surprises. There are some questions about neuroscientific research activities that are out in left field for an understanding of human bonding. Less strange sounding is research on, say, serotonin or the prefrontal cortex or alcohol (the prefrontal cortex has been linked to violent behavior). More strange sounding is the potential from music training and brain workouts, for example. Music training has been shown to upgrade brain circuitry and increase some mental functions. On social neuroscience and human bonding, social work (as suggested in chapter 1) should anticipate the unfamiliar.

Let's return to the Brain Briefing mentioned earlier and to the discomfort of coping with incompleteness. "Give all to love. Obey thy brain," overclaimed the Society for Neuroscience's (2006a) Brain Briefing, because love is about more than the brain. Return to my claim that the analysis of love—or anything else about human bonding in general—should not shift entirely to the province of the biological. Although biological elements such as oxytocin are important in understanding a couple's relationship, so is the contribution of the large literature of thinking about love (e.g., C. S. Lewis, 1960, on the four kinds of love; and Ackerman, 1994, on the natural history of love). Social workers should remember that what is required is a placing of biological or any other data into the perspective of the transactional model. That is, data should be interpreted via the interactions among psychological, biological, social, spiritual, and other domains.

Let's now turn to another link: neuroscience and trauma.

5

Linking to Social Work

Trauma

What is trauma? It is derived from the Greek word for "a wound." It's an emotional or physical wound, such as child abuse, sexual battery, natural disaster (Hurricane Katrina, for instance), domestic violence exposure, repeated foster care placements, bullying, chronic community violence, and other experiences that are typically painful or distressful or shocking. A trauma is a wound that can alter the cells, structure, and functioning of the brain (e.g., shrinking dendrites and decreasing the birth of new cells in the hippocampus; Society for Neuroscience, 2003). It is a wound that can alter brain and body in ways that are challenging for the individual and society. It's a wound that frequently leads to long-term mental and physical effects (e.g., depression, memory problems, posttraumatic stress disorder (PTSD), complex post-traumatic stress disorder (C-PTSD), and affect dysregulation. The effects of the wounding can include altered cardiovascular regulation, behavioral impulsivity, increased anxiety, increased startle response, sleep disturbances, changes in cognition and perception, aggressive behavior, irritability, outbursts of anger, hypervigilance, and restricted range of emotion. It can challenge an individual's ability to cope.

Why should social workers and other human service specialists be interested in the brain's link to trauma-based experiences and behavior? There are at least two reasons why we should focus on such a complex human organ that we don't routinely study or incorporate into our assessments.

Increase Reliance on Science-Based Explanations

First, we should increase our reliance on science-based explanations and decrease our dependence on folk "knowledge"; and we need to do this in a context where the availability of neuroscientific explanations promises to increase significantly in the coming years. It's not that folk knowledge is unhelpful; it's that scientific explanations are more reliable. It's not that we have no scientific explanations beyond neuroscience; it's that neuroscience provides and encourages important scientific explanations.

On the matter of context (just mentioned), it has been only recently that research has pointed emphatically to the dire results of trauma in the brain, and yet the linkage is far from simple. The complexity of such linkage is suggested by the simple fact that what is felt to be traumatic by one person is not necessarily experienced as traumatic by another; experiences affect different people differently. We need to know more about the "why."

On the matter of more science-based explanations, take PTSD as an example. We are not limited to traditional approaches, such as talk therapy. A neuroscience-based approach might recognize the studies of brain chemicals and structures altered in PTSD. An approach might be to target a brain chemical involved in coordinating the body's response to stress, corticotrophin-releasing factor (CRF): "And NIH–funded studies show that drugs called selective serotonin reuptake inhibitors improved the memory of patients with PTSD and reduced shrinkage of brain tissue in the part of the brain involved in memory and emotion, helping PTSD patients better deal with traumatic memories" (Society for Neuroscience, 2006b, p. 1). Preventive measures are also reported (e.g., using beta-adrenergic blockers to prevent the onset of PTSD after a trauma).

We do have useful explanations, some of them the valuable fruits of folk knowledge. For instance, prolonged and repeated experiences of trauma, deliberately perpetrated by people (as contrasted with natural disasters), are generally more difficult to tolerate. The more difficult or traumatic situation is when the wound is deliberately inflicted by a person who is in a relationship with the victim and the victim is dependent on such person (e.g., in a parent-child relationship; Giller, 1999). It is in this sense that Osofsky (2004) refers to trauma as a "family affair."

Yet more extensive neuroscientific and other science-based explanations can help social workers in explaining the emotional, psychological, social, and behavioral difficulties that we encounter. Persons who have endured various social and psychological traumas are frequently found as clients in social service and human service agencies and being served by social workers. Such knowledge can enhance our assessment and intervention efforts. Even more reliable science-based explanations are desirable to help clients manage, prevent, and/or alleviate ensuing problems—client practice-level understandings. They are also valuable for the other levels of understandings—and for the policy-relevant and fundamental understandings—described in chapter 1.

Incidence and Severity of Problems Linked to Trauma

The second reason for focusing on the brain is that the incidence and severity of problems linked to trauma are both large.

Incidence

Note the incidence of childhood trauma. In this, let us include those children who are physically or sexually abused; psychologically maltreated or neglected; those living in the presence of domestic violence; those who experience natural disasters, car accidents, exposure to community violence; and any other event that is life threatening and exposes the child to extreme emotional or physical wounds. In the United States, it is estimated that 3 million children were referred to child protective service agencies in 2004 (U.S. Department of Health & Human Services, Administration for Children and Families, 2004). Thirty percent of these children (872,000) were eventually determined to be victims of child abuse or neglect. Although these numbers represent a decrease in reported victimization over the past 3 years, they do not represent the total picture of children exposed to trauma, because no one is counting those who are exposed to trauma other than child abuse and neglect. It is believed that the numbers of children exposed to extreme trauma is much greater than these statistics show (Weber & Reynolds, 2004). It is also noteworthy that the national data demonstrate that the youngest children (i.e., those in the birth to 3 years category) are victimized at the highest rate and the next highest rate of victimization is among children ages 4 to 7. Many of these children will eventually develop physical, psychological, social, behavioral, and cognitive problems. The type of problem that ensues, and its severity, is dependent on the type of trauma, its intensity and duration, and the age at which it occurred. For example, when the trauma occurs before age 4, it is more likely that the child will develop psychotic or prepsychotic symptomatology. Trauma that occurs after the age of 4 usually results in anxiety and affective symptoms (Perry, 1994).

Take the incidence of PTSD as another example. The Society for Neuroscience (2006b) reports that 5.2 million Americans between 18 and 54 years of age have PTSD every year. Twice as many people in the New York metropolitan area had PTSD, compared with the rest of the country, after September 11, 2001. Some 30% of Vietnam veterans and 8% of Gulf War veterans developed PTSD. Thirty percent of traumatized children develop PTSD (Perry & Ishnella, 1999) based on *DSM-IV* criteria. However, this may be too simplistic an understanding, as persons who have been exposed to repeated and long-term trauma usually meet the diagnostic criteria for many diagnoses; in some situations, the PTSD symptoms are not very evident and may be secondary to other psychosocial and physical problems. Or the person may have what has been described as C-PTSD, which results from extended exposure to prolonged social and/or interpersonal trauma (Herman, 1992). This form of the disorder is seen in situations of incest, child sexual abuse, and domestic abuse and may result in the loss of a sense of safety, trust, and self-worth, and the loss of a coherent sense of self (Herman, 2000).

Severity

On problem severity, consider children of trauma in the school setting. They may have difficulty attending to the teacher; have problems processing, storing, and retrieving information; and experience problems acting in an age-appropriate manner. Their hypervigilance may make them extremely fidgety, and they may have great difficulty even staying in their chairs. Developmental delays in motor, language, social, and cognitive development frequently occur. Maltreated children will also display very immature soothing behaviors, such as biting themselves, banging their heads, rocking, scratching, or cutting themselves. Their emotional functioning is often compromised, which can lead to indiscriminant attachment-like behaviors such as approaching and trying to hug total strangers. This kind of behavior can be understood as the child reaching out to feel safe. Children who are abused or neglected also learn inappropriate modeling from the person who has abused or neglected them, and this sends the message that abusive behavior is appropriate to use with others. This is one of the reasons why sexually abused children are more at risk for future victimization and why sexually abused boys (and occasionally girls) sometimes become sexual offenders themselves. Aggression and cruelty are also frequently seen in neglected and/or abused children.

In a recent study of 17,337 adults, to give another example, eight adverse childhood experiences were assessed as a measure of cumulative childhood stress (Anda et al., 2005). Results showed that as scores increased in the adverse childhood experience domains of abuse, witnessing domestic violence, and serious household dysfunction, the risk of negative outcomes in the areas of affect, somatic problems, substance abuse, memory, sexual behavior, and aggression also increased. In other words, there was a direct relationship between adverse childhood experiences and problematic behavior in numerous domains later in life. Trauma can have lifelong sequelae, affecting many areas of functioning. An example is found among older adults who are seen in hospitals, nursing homes, assisted care environments, and hospice settings.

To increase their reliance on science-based explanations, social workers and other mental health professionals should study trauma in the light of three main understandings. First, these human service workers should examine trauma within a neurodevelopmental perspective, seeking explanations in terms of the growth and functioning of the brain. Second, they should recognize that the biological is important but not *the* decisive determinant, as can be illustrated by considering the significance of a social or other dimension such as that of the caretaker in childhood. Third, there is the advocacy role, especially in identifying and arguing for the kind of neuroscientific research questions that are considered most relevant to challenges in living. The importance of advocacy should be recognized in, for example, identifying less scientifically recognized traumas such as child neglect. This chapter considers each of these three items in turn, but it opens with a case example of one particular "wounded" child.

Darryl: The Quest for Better Social Work Practice

Here's a case example, a kind often enough encountered in social work. Look for instances of the traditional or folk remedy (and nonremedy), instances of remedial help from neuroscientific explanations, and instances of neuroscience serving as a catalyst for expanded treatment services. It is unreasonable to expect, yet natural to hope for, magic-bullet solutions. Yet in the context of a highly productive neuroscience, it is reasonable to be alert to what will transpire and what is most promising.

A 9-year-old American male (we will call him "Darryl") is being seen in a day treatment program located in an elementary school setting. The child has a history of hyperactivity, impulsivity, and mood swings. At school, he is disruptive and defiant; he has frequent temper tantrums and negative peer interactions. He is mostly inattentive in the classroom. Darryl's family history provides some understanding of the trauma he has endured. Both of his parents have been addicted to cocaine, and his mother was recently released from jail. According to case records, the mother used cocaine, marijuana, and alcohol during her pregnancy with Darryl. He has an older brother who also has attention deficit hyperactivity disorder, and both of them live with their grandmother. The day treatment case manager has developed an Individualized Service Plan that includes the following goals: learn appropriate social skills; improve self-control; reduce frequency of temper tantrums, inattentiveness, and hyperactivity; and reduce disruptive and defiant behaviors. The case manager knows that before any treatment goals can be attained, her first task must be to develop a relationship with this child. However, after several weeks of earnest attempts at relationship development, she finds that Darryl still refuses to talk with her about anything at all. Often, he will walk away while she is trying to talk with him. The case manager is severely frustrated, feels incompetent, and is beginning to think that Darryl is incorrigible.

This is the point where we need to look at, and perhaps rethink, how we are conceptualizing this situation, rather than blaming the client for his resistant or bad behavior. Let's use the transactional model and its bio-psycho-social-spiritual domains. As we understand what has probably occurred in Darryl's brain (biological domain), we can begin to see why his seeming unwillingness to engage with another person (the social) is not a conscious choice on his part but perhaps a reflection of his brain being unable to respond. We can assume that Darryl's parents were largely unavailable to him as an infant (the social), due to their drug addictions (the biological), and we must factor in the bio-logical vulnerability he faces as a result of the drugs that were transmitted in utero. Probably he was neglected by his parents (bio-psycho-social-spiritual domains) and therefore did not learn how to regulate his emotions. His mother and father were unavailable emotionally because they were overwhelmed by their own stresses, probably using drugs to calm themselves and burdened by the additional stress of having to maintain a drug habit. As a result, Darryl's right brain (which regulates social and emotional functioning) was unable to interact regularly with the right brain of a primary caretaker who was emo-tionally regulated. The poorly developed right brain would have adversely affected his left brain development, which regulates rational and cognitive processes. Severe, chronic stress has plagued his brain such that a logical response is inhibited; there exists a disconnect between thinking and feeling. In transactional terms, the lack of psychological and social input (from his care-taker) changed the actual structure of Darryl's brain at an early age (probably both in utero and postnatally) and he became poorly attached. This then affected his ongoing development at every stage of life. Now at the age of 9, Darryl is facing life with deficits in his biological domain, his psychological and social domains, and probably his spiritual domain as well. Because each of these individual domains has an impact on every other domain, and each has changed as a result of this interaction, he is faced with a complex array of prob-lems in functioning. Currently, the challenge in living is for the case manager to develop a relationship with Darryl, so that she can affect his ongoing bio-psycho-social-spiritual development.

The case manager's rather traditional approach involved spending time with Darryl. She was trying to involve him in class and group activities, getting him to self-disclose his thoughts and feelings, establishing boundaries, and identi-fying his unacceptable behaviors. Behavioral checklists and consequences were routinely applied.

Turn now to an alternative, developed under the inspiration of neuro-scientific research. To understand Darryl's unresponsiveness, the case manager might use the Stress Model theory of behavior, a novel method developed by social workers Heather Forbes and B. Bryan Post (2006) to work with attach-ment-challenged children and their parents, which provides love, affection, and trust, rather than fear and punishment (see the Web site of the Post Institute for Family-Centered Therapy: www.postinstitute.com). According to the Stress Model, all behavior is derived from a state of stress, and what lies between the behavior and the stress is a primary emotion (either love or fear). To calm the stress and diminish the behavior, one must understand, process, and express the emotion that is primary. In Darryl's case we will assume that the primary emotion that drives him (as is the situation with other children of trauma) is fear. His defiant, impulsive, hyperactive, and angry behaviors are fear based, and they tend to create fear in everyone who comes in contact with him. So the case manager must be in touch with her own feelings of fear, understanding that Darryl's anger and defiance are really coming out of deep-seated fearfulness. Her fearfulness makes the case manager want to threaten or control Darryl, when she needs to look for opportunities to join him emotionally and work on building their relationship. As she begins to understand that Darryl's impulsive and disruptive behavior is his way of communicating underlying fear-based feelings, she can provide a safe emotional space for them to talk about the feelings and what happens within him that causes him to move into a state of fear. It is important for the case manager to work on being present with the child (a challenging task for a chaotic and demanding school environment), by listening to him, connecting with him, and validating what he is experiencing. Even though Darryl misbehaves frequently, it is crucial that the case manager not judge his behaviors and not try to apply logic or reasoning. She should not try to fix the child nor give him directions about how to act differently.

The case manager's main task is to regulate Darryl with her own calm and caring presence. "Protect yourself against your mirror neurons!" she might think. The mirror neuron mechanism is central in learning by imitation. Largely through this mechanism, the brain learns by observing how others behave in different situations. Tancredi (2005) explains that "These (mirror) neurons in humans involve a network which is formed by the temporal, occipital, and parietal visual areas, as well as two additional cortical regions that are predominantly motor" (p. 40). By repeatedly exposing him to her calmness and caring presence, the case manager might hope that the norms of calmness and caring will become wired in Darryl's brain. As Tancredi (2005) indicates, "The mirror neuron system, among other functions, is pivotal to the representation of sequential information, and to imitation" (p. 40).

Working with a child such as Darryl in a school setting can be especially challenging, because the school's behaviorally based approach is counterproductive with a traumatized child and will require ongoing efforts to educate teachers to this new way of intervening. Obviously, the goal here is for Darryl to behave in a more controlled, less impulsive, and more socially appropriate manner. But giving Darryl consequences for inappropriate behavior is punitive and will make him more fearful, because inappropriate behavior is derived from a neurophysiological state of upset or stress, and this needs to be calmed before the behavior can change. Consequences are a way of controlling behavior, but they do not address the underlying developmental problem that is causing the behavior. The misbehaviors should be discussed with Darryl, not to punish and shame, but rather, to try to understand their derivation.

Is it not possible to leverage the availability of more neuroscientific explanation to induce actions that would seem prudent in any circumstances, scientific or nonscientific? Could neuroscientific explanations serve as a catalyst for doing more for Darryl? I think so. Although the day treatment case manager works with Darryl in the school setting, for example, there also needs to be intervention in the home setting. This is often problematic, as school social workers are often not permitted to provide services to the student's family. But if Darryl is to receive the therapeutic services he requires to succeed in elementary school and prevent further severe psycho-social problems in later life, his total caretaker environment must be reeducated. The case manager must help the grandmother to become a significant regulatory figure, by educating her to what Darryl's brain requires to learn to modulate his emotions. Through modeling, his grandmother can teach Darryl how to engage the thinking part of his brain (the frontal cortex) and keep the right side of his brain regulated (i.e., learn to deal with stress so that it is manageable). In addition, it will be helpful, though a tough challenge, for the case manager to educate the school staff and grandmother about positive and negative feedback loops.

A feedback loop describes what occurs between two people (frequently a caretaker and child) that is an unspoken, physiologic communication (Forbes & Post, 2006). It seems that Darryl is frequently caught within a negative feedback loop. So for example, when Darryl becomes upset about a difficult school task and shuts down, becomes passive, and irritable, the teacher also becomes negative and irritable (because she has experienced this many times with Darryl). For change to occur, the negative communication needs to be met with a positive response rather than a negative reaction. We can easily see how difficult this might be for the teacher. A positive response to such a situation might be for the teacher to say, "I can see that you're having trouble with this task; why don't you take a few minutes' break, do some stretching exercises, and then we can try the task again." This kind of response will take the situation into a positive feedback loop, which will be empowering for Darryl. Obviously, this is not easy to do and will require much practice. It also requires that the adult (be it the teacher, case manager, or grandmother) be willing to move from a place of blame to one of understanding. This kind of understanding will encourage Darryl to respond in a positive way, to try to cope with his "wounds."

A Neurodevelopmental View

For social workers and other human service professionals to increase their reliance on science-based explanations, they should examine trauma within a neurodevelopmental perspective. They should seek explanations in terms of the growth of the brain. The ultimate effect of the trauma depends significantly on the child's developing brain and which critical period of development is affected. A critical period is when that part of the brain is organizing and requires specific input at that time to grow normally. This is not to deny that brain plasticity is lifelong. The brain is continually changing in response to cultural and other inputs until the moment of death, as was noted in chapter 3. Yet there are critical periods in brain development.

Let's consider the typical childhood and adolescent brains.

Childhood

The first 3 years of life are crucial in terms of plasticity. This is an especially plastic brain development period, during which persons and events external to the child have a great influence on which neurons and neuronal connections in the brain will develop and which neurons and connections will wither away. The fuller story is more complicated, as even shorter time periods—within the 3-year period—are critical for certain functions (e.g., some language hearing skills).

There are several brain parts that are especially disrupted and changed in these years in the presence of trauma. They are located in brain areas that are involved in our responses to stress and fear. They are the brain stem and locus ceruleus (which regulate homeostasis); the hippocampus, amygdala, and frontal cortex (which form the memory systems and are involved in emotional states and learning); and the orbito-frontal cortex, cingulate and dorsolateral prefrontal cortex (which involve executive functions). The major neuroendocrine stress response system (the hypothalamic-pituitary-adrenal [HPA] axis) is also heavily influenced by trauma. It becomes activated when the body experiences stress. The result is a release of cortisol and adrenocorticotropic hormone, which—as mentioned earlier—helps to manage alarm reactions to stress and enhance survival. Studies show that early life stress, such as child maltreatment, may lead to disruptions in HPA axis functioning, which in turn may result in depression and anxiety disorders among adults (Mello, Mello, Carpenter, & Price, 2003; Van Voorhees & Scarpa, 2004).

Bruce Perry (2004a, 2004b, 2004c), a child psychiatrist who is known for his work on the effects of trauma on children, describes what transpires during these early stages of growth and development and how exposure to traumatic events and experiences can alter the brain. Perry describes a hierarchy of brain organization, which ranges from the brainstem and diencephalon to the limbic area and neocortex. The brainstem is the most basic part of the brain, and it bears repeating (see chapters 3 and 4) that it must be functioning by the time the infant is born, because it regulates heart rate, blood pressure, body temperature, and respiratory functions. Therefore, its sensitive developmental period (i.e., more sensitive to environmental input) is primarily in utero, and insults that occur during the third trimester of pregnancy can adversely affect brainstem functions (e.g., sleep, feeding, self-soothing). The diencephalon, which includes the thalamus and hypothalamus, develops mainly during infancy and is involved with motor regulation, arousal, and appetite and satiety.

The limbic system is more complex than the earlier two brain areas and develops most during early childhood. It includes the amygdala, hippocampus, and basal ganglia. Key functions mediated by this system are memory, emotion regulation, affect regulation, and primary sensory integration. Therefore, a child who experiences trauma at the age of 2, 3, or 4 years may develop problems with memory; ability to regulate emotions; and ability to integrate what he or she hears, sees, feels, touches, and smells. It is likely that the child's emotional, behavioral, and cognitive development will be adversely affected by such traumatic experiences. Studies have found that persons with PTSD (which can be one of the results of childhood trauma) have significantly decreased hippocampal volume (which points to damage in this area), and persons with a history of severe childhood trauma are prone to eventually develop smaller hippocampi (van der Kolk, 2003). Implications of these findings are that the person with damage to the hippocampus may not be able to integrate various sensory inputs; he or she may have problems remembering events within their context and have difficulty learning from negative experiences. For example, a child with hippocampal damage might be prone to show certain emotions in a context that is inappropriate. Does this sound familiar to you? Many of the children we work with in schools and child welfare settings, for instance, seem to have these problems. Other studies demonstrate that hippocampal damage is associated with memory deficits, cognitive impairment, lack of coping responses, and dissociation (Ratna & Mukergee, 1998). It is clear that damage to the child's developing hippocampus will lead to numerous deficits in how the child is able to perform in the school setting.

What exactly occurs within the child's brain in the presence of relational trauma? (see Figure 5.1). By understanding this better, we will be in a stronger position to understand and help traumatized children manage their symptoms more effectively (i.e., their dysfunctional stress responses, emotion-laden behavior, anxiety, irritability, impulsivity, and educational underachievement). The trauma is experienced as extreme stress, and in an attempt to adapt to it, the body engages in two response patterns: the hyperarousal response and the dissociative response (Perry & Pollard, 1998). These stress response patterns are used concurrently or at different times based on age, gender, and nature of the trauma, though they may vary during the child's development and the period of the stress. When a child is exposed to stress or trauma, the usual first response is hyperarousal, an adaptation to threat that allows for the freeze, flight, or fight reaction to occur. In this initial stage of threat, the arousal systems of the brain become activated. The child becomes vigilant concerning his or her surroundings and may start crying or screaming. The sympathetic component of the autonomic nervous system is activated, and this results in increased heart rate, blood pressure, and respiration. Resistance sets in, and the child freezes in place. Defiance is demonstrated and then aggression kicks in so that the child can fight.

In the presence of certain traumas (e.g., child sexual abuse), the immediate response may be dissociation, which allows the child to be detached from what is happening, becoming compliant and numb to the abuse. Perry (2004b) offers specific suggestions for parents, teachers, and others working with traumatized children so that they can provide the kinds of interventions that can quiet and contain the traumatized child who is becoming emotionally unregulated. These suggestions help us to know where the child is on the arousal

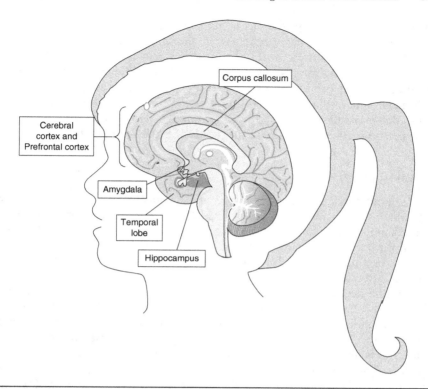

Figure 5.1   Brain Structures Adversely Affected by Child Maltreatment

continuum, whether we should talk to the child or stop talking, and how the child can be calmed (see www.ChildTrauma.org, for specific suggestions). To summarize, traumatic attachments lead to hyperarousal and dissociative responses, which become imprinted in parts of the developing right brain. As a result, the brain structure is changed, and it is thought that this is what leads to inefficient stress-coping mechanisms. These poorly developed mechanisms eventually lead to PTSDs.

In its simplest form, stress can be defined as "anything that threatens an individual's survival" (Sadock & Sadock, 2003, p. 823), or anything that disrupts the homeostasis of body systems. The individual's response to stress concerns what will lessen the stressor's impact and restore homeostasis or equilibrium. The body's "fight or flight" response when exposed to a real or perceived danger leads to reactions in the brain, the autonomic nervous system, the HPA axis, and the immune system.

In the presence of trauma, the child's brain is activated by a state of fear. In this stressful situation, the child feels that his or her survival is threatened and thus engages in a "fight or flight" reaction. To survive, the child must modify his or her emotions, behavior, and thinking to adapt to the threat. This adaptation helps the child to manage the threat, but if the threat persists, the chronic fear state becomes maladaptive, resulting in the child becoming hypervigilant, exhibiting increased muscle tone, focusing on threat-related cues, feeling anxious, and behaving impulsively. These reactions and behaviors are necessary while the threat persists, but they become maladaptive as the threat ends. Ultimately, the response to extreme stress results in an altered kind of equilibrium that is less flexible and results in great fatigue to the body and its systems. The person survives, but at great cost to his or her overall functioning.

Adolescence

As another case study, let us consider an 18-year-old female (we will call her "Amelia") seen by a clinical social worker. The client complains of feeling anxious, depressed, having relationship problems with her boyfriend, isolating herself from others, and being fearful of negative interactions with others. After several meetings with the client, the social worker learns that Amelia has a history of attention-deficit disorder, anorexia, bipolar disorder, and has been chronically neglected by her parents; the client was physically abused by her father before he left the home when she was 2 years old. She also reports that she drinks alcohol to excess and has a history of cutting herself on her arms and stomach, so as not to feel emotional pain. This girl does not meet any of the specific criteria for PTSD, but she certainly appears to have been traumatized, very possibly is attachment challenged, and appears to use the adaptive response of dissociation. She always dresses in black; she has a very flat affective quality and is monosyllabic in her verbal responses. The effects of the early trauma endure.

Notice how early trauma can affect this crucial adolescent stage of development. Development of a child occurs via a sequential process, in which each stage of development builds on the earlier stage. Therefore, when trauma occurs at one period, its effects typically are carried over into the next period, where the problem is compounded by the new demands of the next stage. This is why trauma that occurs at the earliest stage of development, or over an extended period of time, is likely to result in generalized and serious difficulties throughout a person's life. Studies have found that functional deficits in the brain's prefrontal area, among persons with a history of childhood trauma, are related to antisocial and aggressive behavior during late adolescence (van der Kolk, 2003). Each of these brain regions builds on the other in a hierarchical way so that earlier brain areas that are negatively affected by trauma transmit the damage to later developing areas that build on the earlier ones. This is why trauma experienced at an earlier age is cumulative and therefore likely to result in more serious forms of psychopathology, including multiple diagnoses of mental disorders. If the early trauma is not recognized by the clinician, misdiagnoses and misguided treatment may result.

As noted in the previous subsection, the brain is at its most plastic during infancy and early childhood, meaning that it is most receptive to environmental input during these times. As a result, the infant or young child is most vulnerable to experiences (be they nurturing or neglectful) during these very early years. The brain is central to what we are discussing here, but we need to keep in mind that the brain develops based on messages that are encoded in our genes, and most genetic information interacts with life experiences. The timing of the trauma has great impact on the child's developing brain and how it might be damaged. If at all possible, it is important to determine when the traumatic events occurred (i.e., immediately following birth, during infancy, early childhood, or school age). Being able to locate the trauma in time, and determining whether it has occurred chronically, is an important part of an assessment process.

Returning to Amelia, we find that in addition to the numerous psychiatric problems that this late teen is struggling with, her brain has not fully matured. Although adolescents sometimes behave as if they were adults and though it used to be thought that their brains were fully developed, recent studies have found that adolescent brains are not yet fully mature. Adolescent brains are still growing and continue to become more efficient into their 20s. Researchers at the National Institute of Mental Health and the University of California Los Angeles conducted a 10-year study in which they used magnetic resonance imaging to scan the brains of 13 healthy children every 2 years, to see how the brain develops (Gogtay et al., 2004). There were many significant findings, but one of the most interesting was that the prefrontal cortex, which is responsible for planning, judgment, and self-control, is one of the last brain parts to mature. (This is part of the neocortex, along with the frontal, temporal, and parietal lobes, and the corpus callosum. The neocortex is implicated in abstract and concrete thought, language, reasoning, problem solving, self image, and socialization.) The prefrontal cortex does not fully develop until late adolescence or young adulthood.

Prior to the publication of some recent studies, it was generally believed that by the age of 16 years, a child's frontal cortex had matured (Sowell, Thompson, Holmes, Jernigan, & Toga, 1999), but we now know better. A 16-year-old adolescent may still be unable to make good executive decisions or be planful. Added to this is the finding that gray matter in the brain (working tissue of cortex) is overproduced during the first 18 months of life, and then excess is discarded and again overproduced just prior to puberty. Again, there is a pruning of the overproduced gray matter, so that during adolescence, the brain circuits that are not used are pruned away or lost (the "use it or lose it" paradigm). The implications are vast. When an adolescent uses drugs or is depressed, for example, the result can be actual brain damage caused by loss of neuronal matter. Adolescence is obviously a significantly plastic period for brain development, and this could be taken advantage of positively by parents, teachers, and society.

As an aside, the Gogtay et al. (2004) participants, when compared with data from Alzheimer's patients, showed that the brain areas that matured last in youth (those that provide executive functions) were the first areas to lose function in dementia. The parts of the brain that develop early in childhood (i.e., those that control vision and sensation) do not deteriorate until the end stages of Alzheimer's disease. There seems to exist a total age reversal process in brain development.

Returning to Amelia, it becomes more understandable why she has such trouble regulating her emotions, controlling some of her behaviors, and using good judgment (e.g., in choice of friends and boyfriends); her prefrontal cortex is still immature. These are areas in which she will need much additional assistance, and the research results can be used to lessen her guilt about having made so many bad decisions. As social workers (and parents), it is extremely useful to keep in mind that there are probably some behaviors that a teen cannot control without some help, that they just don't yet possess the brakes to slow down emotions. A related finding is that the amygdala (which serves as a gatekeeper for the emotions) becomes fired up by the release of adolescent hormones during and after puberty. The result is that younger teens were found to make much greater use of their amygdala, whereas older adolescents and adults use the amygdala plus their prefrontal cortex much more. The meaning of this is that adolescents view things differently than adults do, and they are more likely to be influenced by emotion than by the still maturing executive part of the brain ("New Research," 2004). Although the first 3 years of life are critical for brain development, we should not forget that in important ways, the next 16 years are also crucial (Giedd, 2006).

A Multidimensional View

As they increase their reliance on science-based explanations, social workers and other mental health practitioners should recognize that the biological is important but not *the* decisive determinant. In studying trauma, we should always remember that all such issues implicate not only biological but also psychological, social, spiritual, and other dimensions. The biological is critical but does not provide the only source of information, as illustrated here by returning to the matter of the caretaker. All the dimensions, as discussed in chapter 3, interact. It also should be noted however, that some mental disorders (e.g., autism, schizophrenia, and bipolar disorder) do carry a much heavier biological load than others do (Torrey, Bowler, Taylor, & Gottesman, 1994).

Social workers should go further, noting that it would be overly simplistic (and inaccurate) to assert that trauma leads to problems. There exists a much more complex interplay of biological, psychological, social, and spiritual variables that lead to challenges in living. Part of the biological involves structural and functional aspects of the brain that predate the traumatic event(s) and serve as risk or resilience factors for later development. For example, a recent study examined 49 Vietnam veterans and their identical twins who demonstrated minor neurological abnormalities. It found that the twins were more likely to experience PTSD, whether or not they had been in combat (Gurvits et al., 2006). These results suggest that the brain deficits predated the emergence of PTSD symptoms and may predispose the person to such. So we are left with the compelling question (a "chicken or egg" dilemma) of whether trauma leads to problems, whether neurobiological deficits make one more susceptible to trauma, or if there is some complex interrelationship among all of these variables. I suspect it is the latter.

Social workers know that it is false to assume that all children subjected to a particular trauma will look the same or behave in the same way. Thus, they will need to perform a full bio-psycho-social-spiritual assessment on each child. And of course, they must also gather as much information as possible about the child's current functioning in all venues, as well as the family composition and functioning, to include community and family supports or their lack. Using the transactional model will help with this task.

Example of the Caretaker

The quality of the relationship with the caretaker is typically a matter not only of the biological but also of the psychological, the social, and the spiritual. It is a critical determinant of healthy human development and yet not solely a biological determinant. Enter the bio-psycho-social-spiritual perspective.

The body's stress response system, the HPA axis, is reported to be heavily influenced by mother-infant interactions early in the child's life (Hofer, 2003). Hofer's research is based in part on experiences during World War II, when children were evacuated from London to the countryside to escape the bombings. Yet it was found that the evacuated children experienced much more stress and distress than the children who remained in London with their mothers, even though they had to endure tremendous devastation. A mother's presence apparently provided a buffering effect, which led to resilience and ability to manage the stress. This was opposed to separation from mother, which led to a rupture of the attachment bond and loss of physical regulatory mechanisms that the relationship with mother had provided. Putting these results in brain terms, we would say that when mother and infant are interacting, the infant's HPA responses to stress are reduced. But when mother and infant are separated, there is a hyperresponse of the HPA system. Hofer's research provides some beginning understanding of why it is that separation from the parenting figure can be traumatic. It illustrates the significance of nonbiological dimensions.

The social dimension has a significant impact. We have talked much about the attachment bond between the infant and the primary caretaker and how important this relationship can be for future relationships; social workers encounter numerous situations where attachment is less than optimal. The nature of the attachment behavior by the caretaker is clearly conditioned by social factors, and faulty attachment is not always the result of abuse or neglect by the caretaker. For example, frequently the attachment relationship is weak due to parental ignorance about child development or other life stresses that impair the caretaker's ability to provide finely attuned parenting. Just as stress can have a huge impact on the developing fetus, neonate, and young child, so too can it adversely affect the child's parents and caretakers. For example, if a family lives in poverty in a high-crime neighborhood or if a mother is depressed, the chronic stress level within the family will increase and makes it much less likely that the parent will be able to attend to the infant or young child in the all-encompassing way that is required for healthy development. Take the example of adolescent parents, who perhaps have been thrown into motherhood and fatherhood before they are prepared; or who may even count on parenthood as a pathway to love, caring, and a significant relationship. Without assistance and support, such parents may be unable to provide the kind of age-appropriate nurturance and attention that infants require. Adolescent single parents may treat their young children as playmates or friends. Based on inadequate knowledge of childhood development, they may treat their children as if they were adults, with all the expectations included. Traumatic attachments can also be transmitted from one generation to the next, just as other parenting behaviors are passed on from parent to child.

Yet the determinant is not merely social, any more than it is merely biological. For example, recall the insecure-disorganized-disoriented attachment, type D of the four Strange Model attachment categories described in chapter 4 (Ainsworth, Blehar, Waters, & Wall, 1978; Main & Solomon, 1990). Children in this fourth category have endured repetitive and sustained emotional abuse, frequently in their first 2 years of life and are more at risk for mental disorder later in life (especially implicated are dissociative disorders). Yet we know that insecure-disorganized-disoriented attachment is associated with parents who were also victims of abuse.

Furthermore, Schore (2002) describes how the various forms of traumatic attachment lead to deficits in the body's ability to modulate stress, which eventually leads to poor or nonexistent coping abilities. All of this is related to the development of the right brain, which is in a critical growth period during the same time that the infant and the caretaker are developing an attachment relationship. If the attachment is traumatic, there is a huge negative impact on the right brain, which leads to serious vulnerability for this part of the brain and its ability to function effectively. A diagnosis of PTSD is a serious future possibility. The right brain represents the center for dissociation, withdrawal, and avoidance, but it is also the place where the internal working model of the attachment relationship is laid down. In other words, the blueprint for the child's original attachment relationship is located within the right hemisphere of the brain and becomes part of the child's memory system. Children who fall into the Type D attachment category exhibit negative physiological and behavioral changes (e.g., higher cortisol levels and higher heart rates than other attachment categories). They also demonstrate low stress tolerance and are frightened by the parent instead of feeling safe in the relationship with the parent.

Advocating

In increasing reliance on science-based explanations, the social worker and other clinical practitioners should recognize their importance, especially as an observer of challenges in living. On behalf of persons experiencing challenges in living, the social worker has a critical function in advocating appropriate research questions for neuroscience. This role of advocating kinds of research questions is presently being done by groups such as social neuroscientists, neuro–political-scientists, and neuroeconomists (as discussed in chapter 1). Each of these groups has genuine interests that differ from, for example, the cell biologist and each other; they want their research questions addressed in ways that are most relevant to their disciplines and interests. Let's consider an example from neuropsychiatry. Modell (2003) is interested in advocating research questions that speak to the neuroscientific generation of meaning. He claims that metaphors are not just figures of speech. Rather, they are neural substrates for generating meaning. Such generation of meaning is not the same as processing information. It's the way in which metaphor is basic for the brain's understanding of its environment. He discusses his view of how metaphor is the brain's primary mode of understanding and remembering the world. He writes of metaphor in corporeal imagination in terms of transferring between dissimilar domains (e.g., between past and present, and—as in synesthesia—hearing colors and seeing sounds). Modell (2003) also claims that "the metaphoric process (in a brain can be) foreclosed or frozen" by trauma (pp. 40-41). An example he gives is of a person who, having experienced a childhood trauma, experiences great stress as an adult when encountering a parallel kind of activity; in respect to this particular experience, as Modell puts it, "the distinction between past and present was obliterated."

Example of Child Neglect

Although it is generally assumed among neuroscientists that trauma that develops as a result of child physical, sexual, or emotional abuse has detrimental effects on the developing brain, there is less understanding of the role that neglect can play in child and brain development. Child neglect is an issue for which social workers are well positioned to advocate for neuroscientific research, because they so frequently encounter such challenges in living among clients they meet. I am not suggesting that all neuroscientists have neglected child neglect; for instance, Perry (as discussed below) has done important work, but he is one of the relative exceptions.

Neglect has been underemphasized in neuroscientific research because it is especially difficult to define and document. It often goes unnoticed because it can be difficult to detect. Yet social workers know that it is widespread, and it is an example of a research area that needs advocacy. It is usually classified into four broad areas: physical, emotional, educational, and medical; and it tends to occur in a chronic pattern. Of the children who were found to be victims of child abuse or neglect in 2004, more than 60% were neglected by their parents or other caregivers (U.S. Department of Health & Human Services, Administration for Children and Families, 2004). Although this statistic is astounding, it does not necessarily point to an overabundance of ill-intentioned parents;

rather, it is a societal issue. As Perry (2004a) notes, neglect of children is more likely due to parents and caregivers who are ignorant of child development, overwhelmed by other life circumstances, and/or severely distressed. This is why it is extremely important that social workers and others who work with children and parents are well educated about child development (i.e., what specifically a child requires at each stage of development) and can educate parents about what is needed and why this is so important for healthy development. Because children do not grow up in a vacuum, we also need to help parents negotiate the wider environment and access the resources they require to provide their children with age-appropriate care. Beyond this, as suggested, social workers need to advocate for inclusion on the neuroscience research agenda. We have important things to say about child neglect.

Children who experience neglect early in life frequently do not thrive, as social workers and other health and mental health professionals know well. In the early years of the 20th century, for example, it was found that infants who became orphans and were institutionalized prior to age 1 (where they suffered physical and emotional neglect) died at a high rate. Deaths were caused by infections or failure to thrive, which is related to negative attachment experiences. In the 1940s, Spitz found that institutionalized children who survived infancy typically had problems with behavioral and emotional regulation and demonstrated severe social development deficits (De Bellis, 2005). For that matter, 19th-century novelist Charles Dickens was quite aware of some damaging effects of child neglect. Asks his character Oliver Twist, "Please sir, may I have some more?"

In recent years, we have learned much from the experience of Romanian orphans (a topic first mentioned in chapter 4), children who were removed from their parent(s) and placed in state-run institutions during the authoritarian regime of President Nicholai Caecescu. These children began to be adopted by Europeans and Americans (in the 1980s), and they have been studied extensively. Findings provide additional information about the devastating effects of extremely neglectful conditions on the development of infants and young children. These children were placed in orphanages with few staff (e.g., a staff-child ratio of 1 to 60), a lack of tactile and emotional stimulation, and inadequate medical care and nutrition. Studies conducted when these children were at age 3 found delays in physical growth (e.g., smaller body size and head circumference), motor delays, poor social skills, and cognitive and language development delays (De Bellis, 2005). Other study results—of Romanian children adopted by families in the United States and Great Britain—found inattention, overactivity, attachment disorders, autistic-like behaviors, and problems in social functioning.

All of these deficits were found to be associated with the length of time the child was institutionalized. For example, orphans who were adopted prior to age 2 demonstrated increases in IQ and improvement in emotional and behavioral functioning. Those who were adopted prior to age 6 months had made even greater improvements in all areas, when evaluated 4 years after being placed in stable and loving homes (Rutter & English and Romanian Adoptees study team, 1998). Studies conducted in the United States by the Child Trauma Academy have also found improvement in IQ (often as much as 40 points), and the seriousness of developmental delays is directly related to the time the child spent in a neglectful environment (Perry, 2002). Other studies have shown that in situations where children are exposed to physical and emotional neglect that is less severe, there are no significant delays in cognitive or language development, but emotional regulation continues to be problematic (Tizard & Ree, 1974). These research results have serious public policy implications. Clearly, infants and children who must be placed in institutions are more likely to develop in a healthy way if they are kept in the institution for the briefest period of time possible and if the institutional caregivers provide tactile and emotional stimulation as well as adequate nutrition and medical care.

Neuroscience can say more about the effects of neglect on the child's brain and body. In neurodevelopment terms, neglect is defined more specifically as occurring when certain neural systems in the brain are deprived of critical kinds and amounts of stimulation and therefore cannot develop normally (Perry, 2004c). Because we cannot see neural systems with the naked eye, neglect cannot be seen; but its results are observable. Neglect has been studied indirectly through animal studies and more directly by looking at children who have been severely neglected, as in the Romanian orphans just noted. Also recall the discussion in the earlier section on the neurodevelopmental perspective, indicating that child development occurs via a sequential process, in which each stage of development builds on the earlier stage. As was indicated, when neglect occurs at one period, its effects are carried over into the next period, where the problem is compounded by the new demands of the next stage. Therefore, the family relationship experiences that a child has in early childhood are especially significant. To be able to determine the why and how of infant neglect, we need to be able to understand the complex interactions between genetic makeup, psychosocial environment, and critical periods of vulnerability for and protection against maltreatment. Research in this important area, which is called "developmental traumatology research," is only in its beginning stages (De Bellis, 2005).

Preliminary neuroscientific research shows that neglect results in deficits in prefrontal cortex functioning (i.e., attentional and social deficits) and executive functioning (i.e., abstract thinking and everyday memory). The chronic stress of being neglected also increases the activation of catecholamines such as norepinephrine and dopamine, which has the effect of turning off the ability of the frontal cortex to inhibit the functioning of the amygdala (De Bellis, 2005; van der Kolk, 2003). As a result, it is thought that the child or adult will have problems regulating his or her emotions and difficulty inhibiting impulsive behaviors.

There are also some preliminary data to suggest that specific brain impairment (in the amygdala, superior temporal gyrus, and prefrontal cortex) may be related to the problems neglected children frequently have in social relationships (i.e., problems in the development of theory of mind), also known as social intelligence. If this proves to be the situation, we will be much better able to understand why a neglected child has difficulty interpreting the behavior of other people, especially related to what they are thinking or intending. Other brain structures may also be impaired in neglected children, including the corpus callosum, connecting the right and left hemispheres (De Bellis, 2005).

Perhaps what is most striking about the adverse effects of neglect is that children who are neglected early in life continue to have smaller brains as they develop, with fewer cells and fewer connections between cells than do other children. Their brains are less complex, and they experience more problems: they are angrier, more easily frustrated, less able to problem-solve, have decreased impulse control, and lower self esteem (Perry, 2004c). Examples of such early and severe neglect are depicted in Figure 5.2, which shows the brains of "normal" 3-year-old children and that of 3-year-old children who experienced severe neglect.

With their access to challenges in living, social workers are in a good professional position to see the complexities that surround traumas and neglect. Take as an illustration the possible trauma, for children and adults, of immigration. For example, there are the mainstream myths that all immigrants immigrate for a better life and that they must be happy in their "better" lives. Wexler (2006), on the other hand, speaks of homesickness that could be so strong that the "adjustment is fundamentally similar to recovery from bereavement" and that immigrants, and therefore immigrant children, "experience substantial problems moving from one culture to another. Their homesickness and culture shock can be so strong as to make the familiarity of even former unhappiness seem preferable to their current dilemmas" (p. 183). Social workers engaged in communities where there is a multiplicity of kinds of immigrants from various countries of origin can be expected to be more sensitive to such traumatic issues than, for example, neurobiologists might be.

Neuroscientists have paid significant attention to stress and the brain (e.g., in animal studies). Our brain stress system activates several biological mechanisms to facilitate coping by increasing strength and energy. For example, the hypothalamus—as mentioned (see Society for Neuroscience, 2003)—releases the hormone CRF and increases defenses. Traveling to the pituitary, the CRF releases adrenocorticotropic hormone, which heads to the adrenal gland and causes the release of cortisol, yet another hormone. The latter provides energy to deal with the stress; this alerts the person to deal with the perceived danger. There is more than one neural pathway, as discussed in chapter 4. (It was pointed out that another pathway leads milliseconds later through the sensory cortex to awareness; deciding that the perceived danger is not a real danger, the person can stand down from alert status.) Ongoing stress, on the other hand, can negatively affect the brain. Examples of such early and severe neglect are depicted in Figure 5.2. The stress system becomes out of balance. To change the metaphor, the brain setting is maladjusted.

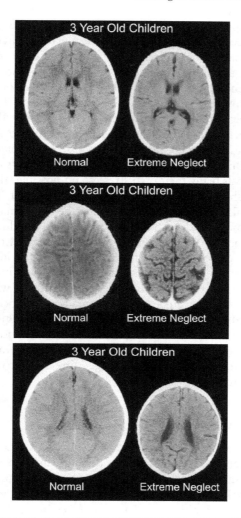

Figure 5.2   Neglect: How Poverty of Experience Disrupts Development. These images illustrate the negative impact of neglect on the developing brain. The CT scans on the left are from healthy 3-year-old children with an average head size (50th percentile). The images on the right are from a series of three 3-year-old children following severe sensory-deprivation neglect in early childhood. Each child's brain is significantly smaller than average and has abnormal development of cortex (cortical atrophy) and other abnormalities, suggesting underdevelopment and maldevelopment of the brain.

SOURCE: These images are from studies conducted by a team of researchers from the ChildTrauma Academy led by Bruce D. Perry, M.D., Ph.D.

It can be assumed that the traumatized child has endured one or perhaps chronic experiences of extreme danger and fear. The frightening feelings that result cannot be handled by the child but are stored in the cells of his or her body. This leads to a child, geared up for survival, who feels unsafe and constantly threatened (Forbes & Post, 2006; van der Kolk, 2003). Therefore, the first task is to provide a safe, predictable environment. The helping person needs to be self-regulated so that this trait can be transmitted to the child who can begin to attach to a regulated figure. Being regulated means being able to experience stress while keeping one's level of stress tolerable; to be calm (Forbes, 2006). This is no easy task, because social workers and other human service professionals bring their own stresses and possible traumas to the professional relationship. However, this needs to be considered. If the helper is not well able to modulate his or her own emotions, he or she may not be the most appropriate person to work with a traumatized child or adult. This work cannot be classified as short-term treatment, no matter what third-party payers might expect. It requires a long-term commitment to provide a child with the enriching and nurturing experiences that he or she has lacked.

Traditionally, traumatized children have been treated with talk therapies and medications, including play therapy, small-group social skills training, behavioral rewards, parent education, and parent training. Recent neuroscience knowledge points to the need for more focused and careful interventions to begin changing the child's neurobiological systems that have been damaged. Social workers should help in suggesting research questions that will yield more finely tuned remedies.

Deeper Than It Need Be

Let's summarize! To increase our reliance on science-based explanations, social workers should examine trauma within a neurodevelopmental perspective, seeking explanations in terms of the growth of the brain. They should recognize that the biological is important but not *the* decisive determinant, as can be illustrated by the significance of the caretaker in childhood. Recognizing their importance as an observer of challenges in living, they should advocate for the specification of appropriate research questions for neuroscience.

Why should social work and other human service specialists be interested in the brain's link to trauma-based experiences and behavior? First, we should increase our reliance on science-based explanations and decrease our dependence on folk knowledge; and we need to do this in a context where the availability of neuroscientific explanations promises to increase significantly. It is also necessary if we are to aim for client practice-level, policy-relevant, and fundamental levels of understanding. Second, the incidence and severity of problems linked to trauma are large. The wound is deeper than it need be.

Let's now turn to another link—to neuroscience and psychotherapy.

6

Linking to Social Work

Psychotherapy

Neuroscience promises to transform both psychotherapeutic under-standings and the practice of psychotherapy; it promises to enrich understanding and practice in clinical social work. Understanding will be deepened over time as the artificial and counterproductive character of the distinction between mind and brain is increasingly recognized in terms of treating mental illness. Practice will be strengthened as the interaction between psychotherapy and the brain is more widely and deeply understood. Psycho-therapy can change the brain, just as the brain can set the parameters of psychotherapy. This interaction is unsurprisingly a powerful corollary of the plasticity of the brain. There is every reason to anticipate that psychotherapies and clinical social work will be enhanced to the extent that brain functioning is appreciated and incorporated into practice. The evidence from neuroscience is significant and compelling.

None of these claims is to denigrate the significant achievements of psy-chotherapists and clinical social workers to date. Social workers frequently feel that the psychosocial work they are doing with a person is useful and helpful to that person. These feelings are often based on the strength of the profes-sional relationship that has been developed between the client and the clini-cian, and they are justified. I have practiced clinical social work for more than 30 years, with a special interest in persons with schizophrenia. My experience convinces me that psychotherapy can be significantly helpful, but we should continue to seek even more effective approaches and steps from neuroscience.

Let us consider in turn some of the conceptual underpinnings of psy-chotherapy and the use of that knowledge for clinical interventions. The first section of this chapter discusses understanding, beginning with dualism of mind and brain, the neurobiology of psychotherapy, and the relevance to clinical social work. The second section examines promising neurobiological models for psychotherapeutic practice that use neuroscience results in terms of neural growth and integration; and results are demonstrable for such conditions as PTSD. It illustrates the practice significance of recognizing neural substrates of psychotherapeutic change. It discusses the practice relevance of the therapeutic relationship in terms of mirror neurons. Practice will be illustrated with case studies, with clients that I will call James, Theresa, Juliet, and Samson. The third section invites social workers to embrace the opportunities to develop understandings and interventions realistically.

Understanding

The old dualism of mind and brain is antiquated in terms of understanding how to treat mental illness. A synthesis of neuroscience and psychotherapy has already begun, and this can be fleshed out in terms of convergence, plasticity, and the brain impacts of psychotherapy. Such understandings are important to disciplines such as social work.

Mind and Brain

The dualism of mind and brain is indeed out of date for the purpose of treating mental illness. I am not speaking here of the philosophical or ontological question of whether mind or matter is primary. What I am asserting is that the dualism of the biological brain and the psychosocial is antiquated in terms of understanding how we treat mental illness.

Such a rejection of dualism—a rejection of the idea that mind and brain can be separated for the purpose of understanding how to treat mental illness—is supported by research on psychotherapy and its effects on the brain. Eric Kandel, who won the 2000 Nobel Prize in physiology for his finding that experience creates new neural connections in the brain, makes a rather astounding statement about the similarities between psychotherapeutic interventions and psychopharmacological interventions, when he says that the focus is at the same level (i.e., the level of individual neurons and their synaptic connections; Kandel, 2001). We shall see, later in this chapter, that some of the brain changes that result from psychotherapy are the same changes that result from the use of medications (Etkin, Pittenger, Polan, & Kandel, 2005). Nancy Andreasen (2001) concurs, saying that psychotherapy—when it is effective—can lead to changes in the brain, which result in changed ways of feeling, thinking, and behaving. Psychotherapy is a biological process as much as is the use of medications, because both are able to change brain functions. That is, such research supports the idea that, as a matter of treating mental illness, dualism of mind and body doesn't fit the facts.

The human puzzle of the relationship of mind and matter has been a pre-occupation since the dawn of philosophy—and perhaps before. Mind refers to "thinking," "spirit," "soul," or some such equivalent. Matter refers to "body" or "biology" or—especially relevant to our case here—"brain." Some people have opted for the view that what is really real (i.e., as a matter of ontology) as a matter of what is fundamentally real is mind or spirit. The idealists such as Hegel and Plato belong to this category. Others have opted for matter (e.g., Hobbes). Yet others have spoken in terms of dualism, claiming that both mind and matter are equally real. Descartes is often described in such terms. But the philosophical story is not as simple as this. There are varieties of idealism (claiming the primary reality of mind) and varieties of materialism (claiming the primary reality of matter), and philosophers have distinguished different meanings of the terms. Then again, other philosophers have not fitted into such categories. It is my claim that we do not have to settle the philosophical (or ontological) question to come to important and fresh understandings of mind and brain for the purposes of treating mental illness.

Sigmund Freud is a symbol of the desirability of rejecting the dichotomy of biology and psychology when it comes to treating mental illness. Freud's own career is also symbolic of how, because of the lack of development in neuro-science in his time, there has been a sort of historical accident in the separation of psychotherapy from the biological.

Fleshing out the idea of Freud as a symbol of rejecting the dichotomy, there is Freud's 1895/1954 work titled *The Project for a Scientific Psychology*, which was an attempt to blend neurology and psychology. It was not published until after his death, as the content was seen as being too advanced for the times. During Freud's youth in the 19th century, a predominant view was that mind and brain were two dichotomous entities, one being psychological and the other physical. Toward the end of that century (i.e., the late 1800s), new knowledge about the brain emerged, including the discovery of neurons and synapses. Sigmund Freud, who by this time had been trained as a neurologist (i.e., one who treats diseases of the brain and nervous system), also had great interest in the mind, and he wanted to combine a psychological view of the person with an understanding of the nervous system. To pursue this interest, he went to Paris to study with Jean-Martin Charcot, who was using hypnosis to treat patients with hysteria to demonstrate the interactions between the body and the mind.

Let's consider the idea of Freud as a symbol of dualism in the historical development of psychotherapy (i.e., of the focus on mind in psychotherapy) as a sort of historical accident. The lack of scientific knowledge about the brain and a very conservative medical establishment led Freud to relinquish his study of the neurobiological and instead focus on the mind. Yet as he developed his theory of personality and the psychoanalytic method, he always hoped for a reuniting of psychoanalysis with its neurobiological base.

In important ways, Freud's vision is being increasingly realized today. Cozolino (2002) is among those who have pointed to such a reuniting of psychoanalysis with its neurological base. Schore's (1994) work, *Affect Regulation and the Origins of the Self: The Neurobiology of Emotional Development,* is seen as a bridge (discussed later) between attachment research, neurobiology, and psychoanalysis, which have been disparate disciplines since Freud's time. The lack of communication between these disciplines and their adherents resulted in a lack of interdisciplinary integration that impedes clinical work (Moskowitz, Monk, Kaye, & Ellman, 1997). This is indeed changing, with the formation of interdisciplinary work groups around the world, where neuroscientists and psychoanalysts can share ideas. In 2000, the International Neuropsychoanalysis Society was founded in London. Its mission is "to promote inter-disciplinary work between the fields of psychoanalysis and neuroscience" (International Neuropsychoanalysis Society, 2008). The society holds an annual congress and publishes the journal *Neuro-Psychoanalysis.*

So does all of this point to a joining of mind and brain, of psychology and neurology? Some people in once disparate disciplines are now talking and thinking together, but there continues to be much discussion within such disciplines about the two concepts of mind and brain. These are complex entities. Although the brain is a physical entity, something with much that can be seen and touched, the mind appears more elusive, as if it were something that must be imagined. Mind is often described as referring to human consciousness, which (in one view) originates in the brain but is manifested in thoughts, feelings, perceptions, emotions, will, memory, and imagination. Mind is often seen as the seat of reason, intention, and desire. Vaughan (1997) believes that it is mind that makes each of us a unique person, as it represents our collected thoughts, feelings, memories, and experiences of the world.

A more expansive conceptualization is that the mind is located at the interface between human relationships and the structure and function of the brain (Siegel, 2001). This "interpersonal neurobiology" allows us to see development as taking place within a social world that interacts with brain function and results in the development of mind. It is in this sense that the mind is understood as being more than the product of the functioning brain; it is also what occurs between brains, via the flow of energy and information (de Kroon & Zammit, 2003). To see this in another way, mind can be understood as growing out of the neural connections of the brain, which have been shaped by human relationships. This conceptualization also is consistent with the way that good relationships with others can nurture and heal the mind (Solomon & Siegel, 2003).

For some, mind and brain continue to be dichotomous entities. Mental health professionals, patients, and their families discuss medication versus psychosocial interventions, as if only one of these interventions is needed (drugs to treat brain illnesses and psychotherapy to treat mental illnesses). Many mental health consumers these days vigorously talk about their brain illness. Although the idea of a mental illness being a brain disease may diminish stigma, it misses what can be called the mind components of illness. The health care insurance industry also uses the mind and brain dichotomy as a rationale for denying equal benefits for mental illness as for physical illness. This lack of parity in health coverage discriminates against persons with mental illnesses and in a sense implies that these illnesses are "all in one's mind" rather than in the brain (i.e., in the body).

For the purposes of treating mental illness, it is worth repeating that mind versus brain (i.e., mental vs. physical, psychological vs. biological) is an outdated dichotomy. Andreasen (2001) points out that this antiquated dichotomy leads to the frequently made distinction (just noted) between medications and psychotherapy. But increasingly psychotherapeutic interventions and psychotropic medications are being combined, and this is being seen as the most effective approach for many mental disorders. Andreasen argues that brain and mind are inseparable and refer to the same thing or activity. "The mind is the product of activity occurring in the brain at the molecular, cellular, and anatomical levels" (p. 27).

Neurobiology of Psychotherapy

There is a convergence between mind and brain and the beginning of a synthesis of neuroscience and psychotherapy, as current research seeks to determine how the mind and brain change as a result of the psychotherapeutic process. Based on the brain's plasticity, the psychotherapeutic process functions as a major form of environmental input and can influence various mind and brain systems, specifically learning, memory, and emotion. Specific experimental results are available about what takes place in the brain during psychotherapy. For example, network integration and coordination can be created or restored. These are topics that deserve explanation here.

Convergence. This convergence between mind and brain was encouraged by the burst of research activity that occurred in the late 1970s when CT and MRI scans were first discovered. At long last, it was possible to view the brain noninvasively. In the ensuing years, the technology has been enhanced so that now we have neuroimaging techniques with high spatial and temporal resolution.

These newer scanning machines allow investigators to see deep within the brain and observe details that were not visible a few years ago. For example, recently a new brain area was located, which in the presence of depression showed high levels of metabolic activity. This area, known as *cingulate area 25,* becomes less active after the depression has been treated. This same brain area was also found to be involved in the brains of persons who are at risk for depression based on a genetic variant in the serotonin transporter (Insel, 2006; Mayberg, 2002). This identification of cingulate area 25 is being used by researchers to begin mapping the circuitry of depression. When the circuitry is more fully understood, we will have a much clearer picture of what brain parts (or functions) are responsible for the emotional aspects of depression, for the vegetative aspects, for the sense of helplessness, for the memory problems, and for the loss of vitality. Because each of these aspects may require different interventions, our ability to clearly identify the location of each symptom of depression moves us much closer to a full biological understanding of this illness.

Plasticity. The psychotherapeutic process functions (as noted earlier) as a major form of environmental input and can influence various mind and brain systems, specifically learning, memory, and emotion (Andreasen, 2001). Psychotherapy has been described as a "controlled form of learning," which takes place within a therapeutic relationship (Etkin et al., 2005). It provides a way of learning about oneself, which some researchers say may influence brain structure and function (Kandel, 1998).

As suggested by neuroscience, the process of psychotherapy relies on the brain's plasticity for its effectiveness. With regard to brain plasticity, we earlier (chapter 2) discussed the importance of critical periods in development. Another piece of plasticity is the idea of activity-dependent changes. In psychotherapy, the actual therapeutic encounter can be considered as the activity, and it is this process between persons that leads to changes within the brain. It should be noted here that different parts of the brain are more plastic than others. For instance, cortical areas (that are closer to the brain's surface) are more easily changeable, whereas subcortical areas (deeper within the brain) can only be changed when they are turned on. In other words, these deeper brain areas (the nonverbal, emotional right hemisphere) are plastic to the extent that their neurons are firing.

The learning activity that goes on between client and clinician can lead to a reframing of emotional and cognitive responses, and this reframing is the result of biological activity that has transpired in the brain (Andreasen, 2001); learning is really a form of synaptogenesis in which the brain keeps reshaping and reorganizing itself throughout adulthood and which is enhanced by the psychotherapeutic process. New treatments must also be developed that use our knowledge about the brain's plasticity.

Brain plasticity refers to mind and brain, and for the purpose of the present discussion, I continue to use both terms. Both the mind and the brain are constantly changing as physical and psychological experiences affect our mental functions and states. The "mind," conceptualized as the functional systems of the brain, includes mental activities such as remembering, communicating through language, and focusing one's attention. Each function of the brain can be described as associated (although recall the warning in chapter 2 against confusing category types) with a specific brain part or region (e.g., thinking takes place in the frontal cortex, experiencing emotions takes place in the limbic system, etc.). This has been learned from mapping functional systems using the PET scan and fMRI. Based on brain plasticity, our brains are always undergoing a process of rewiring, and this of course changes our minds.

The process of psychotherapy does indeed rely on the brain's plasticity for its effectiveness. Brain plasticity, it will be recalled, refers to the impact of the physical and psychological environment on how brain neurons relate to each other. Neurons increase in number, decrease in number, and connect with other neurons based on their ability to wire and rewire with each other and eventually form neural networks. This neural plasticity (or ability to change) is regulated by the environment, which also has a large influence on how genes are expressed. To be more precise, we can describe genes as providing a template and a transcription function (Kandel, 1998). The template function, or sequence of the gene, determines how the anatomical structures of the brain are organized and will function, and these are not much affected by the environment. However, the transcription function of the gene directs the manufacture of specific proteins, which form the neural networks and determine the amount of neurotransmitters that will be available to specific brain systems. This transcription function is highly responsive to environmental input (Gabbard, 2000). This then is how we can understand how the psychotherapeutic process may influence the brain's neural networks and production of neurotransmitters.

Brain impacts of psychotherapy. Let's return to the questions of what takes place in the brain during the process of psychotherapy and how psychotherapeutic intervention uses the brain's plasticity to have an impact on a person's functioning.

To answer these queries, we must have some understanding of neural networks, which are organized groups of neurons that perform the work of our nervous system. In the human brain, neural networks are very complex and can include trillions of neurons that are interconnected. The networks encode and organize all of the behaviors we engage in, from basic reflex actions to sophisticated understandings of emotional and political events and experiences. The integration of neural networks is essential for mental health, and psychopathology is seen as being the result of problems with the integration and coordination of neural networks (Cozolino, 2002). This lack of coordination can result from problems in the caretaking relationship of early years, genetic and biological vulnerabilities, and from trauma that is experienced at any time. Later, we will note how dissociative symptoms that result from traumatic experiences are a reflection of the disconnect between neural networks that manage behavior, emotions, sensations, and cognition, and have also been found to predict later PTSD.

Conversely, psychotherapy is a process through which neural network integration and coordination can be created or restored. This is especially crucial (as illustrated later in the case study of James) for the networks that specialize in emotions, cognition, sensations, and behavior.

Although the research on psychotherapy is much less prolific than studies on psychopharmacology of mental disorders, there does exist a beginning literature on the neurobiology of psychotherapy, which describes findings about brain changes that appear to be based on the psychotherapeutic process. The research describes the effectiveness of psychotherapy, follows the course of the treatment, and makes possible determinations about which patients, with which disorders, can benefit from and should receive psychotherapy. Especially good use has been made of neuroimaging techniques in the study of three common disorders: depression, obsessive-compulsive disorder (OCD), and other anxiety states. Because anxiety and depression are the most common mental illnesses in the United States, this is exciting news. It deserves repeating that such research has become possible due to the advent of more sophisticated neuroimaging techniques, developed in the 1990s, which allow for the scanning of a person's brain during the course of psychotherapy and after the treatment is completed.

Several early studies used PET scans to measure basal brain metabolism in persons who have OCD (Baxter et al., 1992; Brody et al., 1998; Schwartz, Stoessel, Baxter, Martin, & Phelps, 1996). In one study, patients had abnormally increased basal glucose metabolism in the caudate nucleus of the brain (the caudate nucleus is part of the basal ganglia, which is involved in motor control and is abnormal in OCD patients) when compared with healthy comparison patients. Following treatment via exposure therapy, or with fluoxetine (prozac), basal glucose metabolism was lowered to a normal level (Baxter et al., 1992). These findings may point to a specific brain circuit that involves the caudate nucleus as being involved in the symptoms of OCD. In another study, conducted by Schwartz et al. (1996), those persons with OCD who responded to behavior therapy demonstrated larger decreases in caudate metabolism than did patients who were not responsive to the therapy. This study, which replicates the previous one, demonstrated that those who responded to psychotherapy had more normal levels of basal glucose metabolism in specific brain parts. Although these studies were not well controlled, they do show that behavior psychotherapy can change certain brain activity (Etkin et al., 2005).

Social phobia, which is another of the anxiety disorders, has also been studied using PET scans. Eighteen persons who had been diagnosed with social phobia were randomly assigned to receive either the antidepressant medication citalopram or cognitive-behavioral group therapy, or were assigned to a wait-list control group. Participants were scanned and regional cerebral blood flow was assessed during an anxiety-provoking public speaking task, prior to the intervention and again after 9 weeks of treatment or waiting time. Results demonstrated significant improvement in both of the treated groups (i.e., citalopram and cognitive-behavior therapy [CBT]) and no changes among the wait-list group of participants. The improvement in symptoms was also seen in those participants who showed on PET scans a decreased regional cerebral blood flow response in the amygdalae, hippocampi, and neighboring cortical areas (Furmark et al., 2002). These are brain regions that are involved in the body's defensive reactions to threat, and it appears that both medication and CBT can have a positive effect on functioning in these areas.

Several other studies (Goldapple et al., 2004; Paquette et al., 2003) have found brain changes related to treatment with CBT. Seventeen persons with a diagnosis of major depressive disorder (MDD) were given 15 to 20 sessions of CBT and monitored via the Beck Depression Inventory and the Hamilton

Depression Rating Scale. None of the participants was taking psychotropic medication. All research participants underwent a PET scan before beginning and after the termination of the CBT interventions. Fourteen participants completed the course of treatment, and all demonstrated significant clinical improvement, as determined by scores on the Hamilton Depression Rating Scale (Goldapple et al., 2004). The PET scans following CBT showed significant metabolic changes, which included increased metabolism in the hippocampus and dorsal cingulate (limbic area of brain) and decreased metabolism in the dorsal, ventral, and medial frontal cortex (cortical areas of brain).

By way of explanation, this might point to increased metabolism in emotional areas of the brain and decreased metabolism in the upper areas of the brain. Participants in this study were also compared to 13 persons with MDD who had been treated with, and responded to, paroxetine. Findings were different when the two groups were compared; paxil-responsive patients showed increased metabolism in prefrontal areas and decreased metabolism in limbic areas of the brain (Goldapple et al., 2004). These results point to CBT as having a direct impact on the neural correlates of depressive symptoms.

In another study of MDD using fluorodeoxyglucose positron emission tomography (FDG-PET), 24 persons with MDD were compared with 16 normal control participants (Brody et al., 2001). All participants underwent scans at the beginning and end of the study. Those persons with MDD were treated with either paroxetine or interpersonal therapy (IPT), depending on the preference of each patient; control participants received no treatment. The participants who received IPT had 12 weekly psychotherapy sessions with a trained IPT therapist, focusing on improvement in the person's social networks and reduction of depressive symptoms. Based on the IPT model, the concentration was on problems in role transition, interpersonal dispute, social deficit, and grief. After 12 weeks of treatment (either medication or IPT), it was found that both MDD subgroups demonstrated significant mean decreases in scores on the Hamilton Depression Rating Scale, whereas control participants had no significant mean change.

Those participants who received the medication showed a larger mean decrease in scores on the Hamilton Depression Rating Scale (61.4%), as compared with the participants who received IPT (38.0%). But it was determined that the paroxetine-treated subgroup was less ill at baseline (Brody et al., 2001). On the PET scans, both of the intervention groups demonstrated decreases in prefrontal and cingulate gyrus metabolism, though the paroxetine group showed bilateral prefrontal decreases and the IPT group showed only right prefrontal changes. Results need to be interpreted cautiously with all of these metabolic studies, however, based on study limitations (i.e., small sample size, lack of randomization).

Although such studies provide a beginning look at specific brain changes that may result from the psychotherapeutic process, there are additional reasons for using neuroimaging techniques to help us better understand emotional and mental illnesses. Different kinds of brain scans can measure the activity and connectivity of brain parts and functions and help us to see interactions between neural networks. In the future, it is expected that neuroimaging methodologies will make possible the grouping of patients into different types of a disorder (Etkin et al., 2005). Although this could have the potential of further stigmatizing those with a mental disorder, what is more likely is that specific therapeutic interventions will be developed to treat specific subtypes of an illness.

We know that there are different types of depression, for example; but what does each type look like based on biological variables? If we can place a person into a specific biological subgroup, we will be better able to determine who can benefit from which therapy. Rather than having to rely solely on a diagnosis, we will be able to use brain scans to depict how a person's brain will process certain stimuli and therefore which intervention will provide a better outcome. This might help to decide whether a person should be given a psychotropic medication or some kind of psychotherapy intervention, and if so, which type of psychotherapy. Brain scans should also be able to help us better monitor a specific treatment and to make it possible to see signs of recovery or relapse prior to behavior or symptom changes (Etkin et al., 2005).

Neuroimaging techniques can also be used to predict outcome. For example, an FDG-PET study of depression found that higher levels of metabolic activity in the anterior cingulate cortex before treatment resulted in a better outcome. These findings have been replicated, and although they were based on pharmacological treatment, it is thought that they will also apply to psychotherapy (Mayberg et al., 1997). In an imaging study of OCD, it was found that lower levels of metabolism in the orbitofrontal cortex before treatment predicted better response to antidepressants but higher orbitofrontal cortex metabolism prior to treatment predicted better response to behavioral therapy (Brody et al., 1998).

These results demonstrate that different metabolic patterns are correlated with different responses to behavior therapy versus medication. At the time of writing, future research is needed that uses neuroimaging techniques to more systematically explore brain changes that occur following psychotherapy, to determine how these biological processes relate to the conscious and unconscious aspects of psychotherapy and how this is related to the way psychotherapy works (Etkin et al., 2005).

Learning about the self may influence brain structure or function. Gabbard (2000) explains that psychotherapy affects the brain and also has a psychological impact; psychotropic medications also affect the brain and have psychological effects. Preliminary research results indicate that psychodynamic therapy may influence serotonin metabolism (amount is normalized via therapy); cognitive therapy influences thyroid hormone levels in those with major depression (Gabbard, 2000); and supportive relationships influence brain functioning among breast cancer patients (Spiegel, Bloom, Kraemer, & Gottheil, 1989). There is much preliminary evidence that what seems to be curative in the psychotherapy relationship is the emotionally charged relationship that becomes reparative.

Relevance to Social Work

Because the neuroscience research we have discussed is related to psycho-therapy, establishing social work relevance requires linking psychotherapy with clinical social work. Let's start with a view of the problem(s) and then see how neuroscience is indeed relevant by noting the research and by reflecting on our own social work experiences.

The problematic. Clinical social work practice has always had a conflicted relationship with psychotherapy. Is it the same as psychotherapy, or is it a kind of psychotherapy that includes working on behalf of clients and their communities to bring about social and psychological change and to increase access to social and economic resources?

There are some social workers who would say that clinical social work is not psychotherapy at all and to use that term does a disservice to clients and the social work profession. For some, even the term *clinical social work* is seen as an attempt to achieve greater status by setting oneself apart from the rest of social work, and it is much too closely tied to the medical model for the term to reflect what a social worker does.

Clinical social work, in my view, is somewhat different from psychotherapy but closely aligned. Clinical social work is direct practice with—and on behalf of—individuals, families, and small groups: The practice goal is to enhance and maintain psychosocial functioning. Practice settings and interventions might include the following: running a group for male batterers who are receiving services within a family service agency; working individually and in groups with teenage youth who have sexually abused others; providing intensive, in-home services to a chaotic family affected by substance abuse and behavioral acting out; helping a person with serious mental illness to gain independent living skills; working within the Veterans Administration to provide clinical services to persons with PTSD; helping a recovering heroin addict to manage his or her addiction and maintain sobriety.

Clinical social work draws from multiple theoretical frameworks and includes the processes of relationship (Goldstein, 2007), engagement, assessment and formulation, intervention, evaluation, and prevention. Central in any such social work framework is a person-in-situation perspective (Ewalt, 1980; Swenson, 1995). Attention to the larger environment (be it family or commu-nity) is a critical element in what distinguishes clinical social work from psy-chotherapy. Yet the National Association of Social Workers' definition of *clinical social work* also includes the terms *psychotherapy* and *counseling.*

Although we will continue to use the term *psychotherapy,* it should be noted that most writers do not define this term. Therefore, as we look at studies that are trying to determine in what ways psychotherapy may change the brain's structure and function, it is frequently not clear what is meant. Clearly, psy-chotherapy is practiced in a large variety of ways and by a varied group of prac-titioners; what is needed is a breaking down of the therapy process into its specific parts. This is rarely done, and so we often do not know what particular aspect of psychotherapy may be effecting the changes. Much of this remains to be elucidated in future studies about the neurobiology of psychotherapy.

Traditionally, psychotherapy was considered to be a long-term therapeutic intervention that focused on the patient's unconscious conflicts and helped the patient to develop insight through interpretation. For some, that theory still holds true. As such, psychotherapy was based on the power of the therapeutic relationship, with a high value placed on transference and countertransference and other concepts that were closely identified with psychodynamic theory.

In the past 20 to 30 years, as increasing numbers of theories have been converted into practice interventions, there are many different models for intervening. Although psychotherapy is still a kind of planned intervention to help alleviate mental and emotional disorders, it may or may not include a focus on unconscious conflicts, and development of insight is often not a primary goal. Furthermore, although the therapeutic relationship remains important in many models of psychotherapy, in brief forms of therapy (which are increasingly popular), it is sometimes an unimportant component.

There is some skepticism about the evidence for the usefulness of clinical work. Evidence-based practice modalities have also become popular in recent years, and although these tend to use quantitative research methods and exclude others, they often focus on cognitive-behavioral techniques and downplay the therapeutic relationship (Goldstein, 2007). Social workers do typically feel that what they are doing is useful to the client, and it bears repeating that these feelings are often based on the professional relationship between the client and the clinician. But feelings are to be distinguished from thoughts or beliefs, and social workers don't necessarily believe that what they are doing is demonstrably effective, because such a belief would require more empirical evidence to be generally accepted. Also, other mental health professionals refer to the controversy that has surrounded psychotherapy and note that some see this kind of intervention as mere "hand-holding" (Gabbard, 2001).

Relevance. Recently, there has been growing empirical evidence for brain changes related to the psychotherapeutic process, and this directly relates to much of the work done by clinical social workers and other mental health professionals. Beyond this, social workers should reflect on their own case experience, much of which has combined psychosocial interventions with the use of psychiatric medications.

There is a beginning literature that demonstrates that a combination of psychotherapeutic and psychopharmacological interventions are required to adequately treat most mental disorders. An example is provided in a recent supplement to the *Schizophrenia Bulletin,* one of the premier journals for research on schizophrenia, which was devoted entirely to the topic of the psychotherapy of schizophrenia (Carpenter, 2006).

Since the discovery of psychotropic medications in the 1950s and the biological revolution in psychiatry (1960s onward), the biological model of mental illness has focused attention on the physical causes of major mental illness, specifically looking at brain structure and function as causative. The use of psychosocial interventions, especially psychotherapy, for major illnesses such as schizophrenia, has been very limited. This supplemental issue of the *Schizophrenia Bulletin* (Carpenter, 2006) demonstrates the sea change that has occurred, especially among psychiatrists and psychologists. Psychotropic medication alone is not considered to be the most effective treatment for schizophrenia, depression, and many of the anxiety disorders. In essence and echoing what was mentioned earlier, the mind and brain dichotomy has been shown to be obsolete for the purpose of treating mental illness, and what is needed is for us to think in terms of mind and brain systems that work together. If we view mind and brain systems as part of the same whole (i.e., the biological-psychological-social-spiritual perspective), we can argue more strongly for the inclusion of both forms of intervention. If medications alone are used, we may be omitting the psychological, social, and spiritual and cultural aspects of a person's being.

Clinical social workers should reflect on their own case experience—a variant of the kind of reflection that Sigmund Freud did on his own cases. That experience should be persuasive enough that much of what we already do as clinicians can readily be understood in neurobiological terms. If we can understand the neural mechanisms that our interventions involve, we can see how our clinical social work can contribute to—and be shaped by—what can be described as network wiring and rewiring. Recall the vast array of interconnections (wiring, as it were) between the brain's 100 billion neurons, described in chapter 2; also recall the discussion above about plasticity.

Consider the case of James, for example. A 48-year-old man, James is in long-term treatment. I used rather traditional social work interventions such as home visits. After he moved into his own apartment, James felt pride in his new home and wanted to share this with me, so he invited me to have lunch at his apartment. He prepared the lunch himself, and we met at his new home. This proved to be a very edifying experience for James, and I was able to provide much reinforcement for his new social and domestic skills. Much later, I realized that this visit to James's home also provided an opening to the nonverbal and healing capacities of the right brain.

Several years later, James's father died, and this followed his mother's death several years earlier. At the time of his mother's death, I maintained the traditional distance between clinician and client, and we talked about his mother's death and its ramifications for him. I did not officially acknowledge the death, and I believe that James wished that I had done so. By the time his father died, I had more knowledge about the neurobiological aspects of the process, and so I asked if it would be all right if I attended the father's funeral. "Yes, I would like that very much," replied James. Following his father's internment, as people gathered near the gravesite, I approached my client and hugged him, saying how lovely I thought the funeral was. Later, he was able to tell me how much he appreciated my attendance at his father's funeral. I am hopeful that my attendance at the funeral demonstrated attunement with James at a deep level and provided a right-brain to right-brain communication (using nonverbal cues) that will enhance neural wiring.

As we think in neuro terms, we begin to see psychotherapy more clearly and more centrally as a relationship between two brains. Just as in the early days of postuterine life, our brain developed in relation to our mother's brain, so later in psychotherapy, growth is determined by brain-to-brain interactions. What the psychotherapist activates, by being in an attuned relationship with the client, can lead to healing and changes in synaptic plasticity. What becomes aroused and what is turned on and firing within the psychotherapy experience is able to grow and change. When the subcortical emotional centers are aroused and the neurons are firing, then there is the possibility for change and growth to occur within the psychotherapeutic experience.

Practice

Promising neurobiological models (or approaches) have been identified for psychotherapeutic practice that use neuroscience results in terms of neural growth and integration (e.g., dialectical behavior therapy [DBT] and mentalization-based treatment [MBT]). The practice significance of recognizing neural substrates of psychotherapeutic change is supported in the research and can be illustrated by a case study of a woman we will call Juliet. There is practice relevance for the role of the clinician in such neuroscientific features as mirror neurons, and this can be illustrated by a case study of a client we will call Samson. These are claims that are explored in the following paragraphs.

Neurobiological Models

Cozolino (2002) posits that any kind of psychotherapy, no matter what type of theory is used, can be successful to the extent that it fosters neural growth and integration—the kind of wiring and rewiring that we just discussed in the case of James and earlier. Six activities are offered for the enhancement of this integration: (a) establishing a safe and trusting relationship; (b) eliciting new information and experiences from the domains of cognition, emotion, sensation, and behavior; (c) activating neural networks that have been inadequately integrated or dissociated; (d) providing affect regulation via moderate levels of stress alternating with calm and safety; (e) helping to integrate conceptual knowledge with emotional and bodily experience via narratives that are coconstructed between client and therapist; and (f) developing a way to process and organize new experiences that can be generalized to life outside the therapy situation.

To achieve these therapeutic activities, the psychotherapist is directed to be conscious about whether he or she engaged in top-down, left-right, or bottom-up integration.

Top-down refers to brain circuits that move from the top of our head (cortex) down to the subcortical areas (limbic system and brain stem) and then return to the top. Integrating these circuits would make it possible for the cortex to process, inhibit, and organize the impulses and emotions that originate in the brain stem and limbic system. This helps to explain why OCD and ADHD are examples of dysregulation of this neural circuitry. Left-right refers to the two hemispheres of the brain and includes cerebral cortex and limbic areas (i.e., thinking and feeling parts of the brain). As an example, left-right integration makes it possible for a person to put feelings into words (i.e., the left side provides grammatical functions and the right side makes emotions possible; Cozolino, 2002).

Traditional forms of psychotherapy (e.g., psychoanalytic, behavioral, and cognitive-behavioral) all share a top-down approach in which higher order functions such as cognition, affect, and behavior are emphasized, and little attention is paid to their emotional underpinnings (Viamontes & Beitman, 2006). Viamontes and Beitman argue that more attention needs to be paid to the bottom-up aspects of psychotherapy, which can be accessed by understanding the brain.

In my view, the top-down, left-right integration that Cozolino (2002) describes, which attends to the horizontal and vertical planes of neural structure, and the bottom-up approach of Viamontes and Beitman (2006) would provide a more complete approach to a neurobiologically based (or a neurologically informed) psychotherapy (see Figure 6.1). If psychotherapy attended to the emotional foundation of the symptoms that clients present, we would need to help clients develop the neural structures that would allow for self-regulation of affect. Many kinds of psychopathology are seen as the result of a failure to regulate affect, which may involve problems in the development or function of the amygdala, hippocampus, prefrontal lobes, problems with neurotransmitters, or connections among certain brain areas (neural network connections). Successful psychotherapy can be conceptualized as helping the client to develop the necessary skills to regulate his or her own affect (Bradley, 2000; Cozolino, 2002).

Applegate and Shapiro (2005) observe that Marsha Linehan's (1993) DBT is based on the intervention strategies that follow from Cozolino's objectives for fostering neural growth and integration. DBT assumes that a person with borderline personality disorder has a fundamental problem with mood regulation, and many of her behaviors are attempts to regulate these intense emotions. Such clients are seen as living in an invalidating environment that negates emotional expressions and does not teach the person how to label and regulate emotional arousal.

In DBT, the clinician builds an alliance with the client, which is then used to validate the client, his or her experiences, and his or her problems. Via the use of behavioral contracting, the therapeutic alliance also provides safety and is used to help the client develop new cognitive and coping skills, to gain control

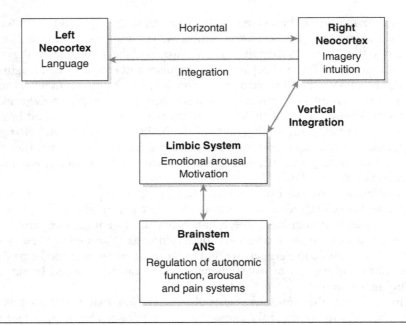

Figure 6.1   Neural Integration (Left-Right, Top-Down, and Bottom-Up)

over mood and to solve problems. These activities can be seen as activating neural networks that lack integration and provide affect regulation. The new narratives that are constructed between the client and clinician assist the client to have a more realistic understanding of others' behavior and respond differently to new interpersonal experiences. DBT has been shown to be effective in several randomized clinical trials of women who had borderline personality disorder and/or substance abuse disorders (Swenson, Torrey, & Koerner, 2002). Although the research on DBT and its efficacy in treating borderline personality and other disorders is still in its infancy, we do know that DBT is widely used. Linehan (1993) maintains that although DBT is not a cure for borderline personality disorder, it is the best treatment that we currently have.

Another model of intervention currently being studied for treatment of persons with borderline personality disorder is MBT. This method of treatment was used in a partial hospitalization program at St. Ann's Hospital, London, and was found to be more effective than the usual treatment. This model used individual and group psychotherapy, and the study concluded that patients' capacity for mentalization was (see the qualification in the next paragraph) increased (Bateman & Fonagy, 2004). Mentalization is the capacity to reflect on and think about one's own feelings and those of others and to be empathically attuned to others. Borderline personality disorder is conceptualized as deriving from disorganized attachment style and unstable emotions and relationships.

MBT is based on a neurobiological understanding of borderline personality disorder, which includes the reward and attachment circuits of the brain (orbitofrontal cortex and nucleus accumbens) and the brain parts and activities involved in disrupted interpersonal interaction. The latter are not fully understood at this time but may involve the anterior cingulate and prefrontal cortex (Fonagy & Bateman, 2006a). The goal of MBT is to enhance or recover one's capacity for mentalization. Fonagy and Bateman also point out that mentalization related to attachment relationships improves only in psychotherapy that is transference focused. Therefore, most aspects of DBT and supportive psychotherapy do not improve capacity for mentalization. On a more hopeful note, Fonagy and Bateman (2006b) conclude that the recent availability of effective interventions leads to greater optimism for improvement and long-term outcomes in the treatment of borderline personality disorder.

Daniel Siegel, who has done much to bring together the fields of neuroscience and clinical practice (Wylie, 2004), also believes that the basic goal of psychotherapy is self-regulation, because in his view, most mental health problems derive from a lack of self-regulation. Siegel uses knowledge of the brain and how it works to educate his clients about the neurobiological components of their illness and to empower them to attain mental equilibrium. For clients who are suffering from PTSD, for example, Siegel explains the difference between implicit and explicit memory, and how these can be understood as being located in different subsystems of the brain. Implicit memory is the first layer of memory to develop, between birth and eighteen months of age, and is unconscious. It includes how-to knowledge, procedural skills, and the emotional and behavioral responses that occur during an experience. Explicit memory develops later and includes actual facts and ideas and what is called "episodic memory" (i.e., the memory of oneself in an episode in the past). What distinguishes these two types of memory is where in the brain they are located, the type of knowledge each forms, and whether the knowledge is retrieved with or without conscious awareness. When we access an implicit memory, we can have a perceptual or emotional response, but there is no sense that this is a memory from the past. Explicit memory involves the hippocampus and higher cortical structures that are able to contextualize the bodily and emotional memories within an autobiographical network.

In PTSD, the frightening memories that are retrieved are thought to be implicit memories; there is no sense that they are coming out of one's past and they are not laid down in words. There is a lack of integration between implicit and explicit, and this lack of memory integration means that the implicit memory has no sense of self or time. It is thought that perhaps the traumatic event, with its huge secretion of stress hormones, temporarily shuts down the hippocampus and its ability to integrate memory (Siegel, 2006). What could bring closure for the person who is suffering from PTSD is being able to reflect on the traumatic experience verbally as a memory of an actual event that occurred in one's past and is now being recalled, rather than a current experience that is felt to be a part of the self and is happening now.

Recognizing Neural Substrates

The therapist should recognize the neural substrates of psychotherapeutic change. Brain networks that organize memory, attachment, emotion, and conscious awareness are particularly relevant for the psychotherapeutic process (Cozolino, 2002). These networks involve the executive brain, which is compared to the CEO of a large corporation, and which organizes relationships among many different neural networks.

The frontal and prefrontal cortices, which manage behavior and emotional functioning, are especially important as they receive a constant stream of sensory, motor, and emotional information from the lower brain parts (i.e., limbic system and brain stem). As this information is received, the frontal areas synthesize it and coordinate actions. The prefrontal cortex is the most forward part of the brain, and just behind it and to the side lie the dorsolateral and orbitofrontal regions. The dorsolateral prefrontal cortex (DPF) is the part of the brain that initially receives the verbal interventions of psychotherapy. The DPF modulates executive functions such as problem solving, organization, working memory, memory retrieval, self-direction, and the use of language to guide behavior. The DPF is said to be where ego would be if we could see it (Viamontes & Beitman, 2006).

The psychotherapeutic process frequently involves helping the person to modulate emotional reactions, which occur largely through the right orbital prefrontal regions. These areas are connected to the anterior cingulate and the amygdala (subcortical structures) and form parts of the emotional network. The cingulate gyrus-nucleus accumbens circuit, where Freud's id might be thought to be located if we could see it, is involved in attaining pleasure and the pursuit of rewards (e.g., chemical dependence), and the nucleus accumbens is the center of the brain's reward system.

The final part of the brain's emotional system is the orbitofrontal-amygdalar circuitry, which could be considered to be the seat of the superego. This circuit moderates the pursuit of pleasure by incorporating the context of the situation, the possible risks, and the potential consequences of behavior. Through its connection to the amygdala, it is involved in emotions that relate to the pursuit of reward and the avoidance of risk. Studies have shown that this circuit can be modulated by the conscious cognitive processes of psychotherapy (Ochsner, Bunge, Gross, & Gabrieli, 2002). For example, by teaching a person how to problem solve and organize his or her world, how to become aware of patterns of behavior that cause problems, and how to modulate emotions, the executive functioning of the frontal cortex can be enhanced and the nucleus accumbens can be tamed. These can be accomplished by strengthening ego. Many of the problems that are brought to the psychotherapy situation are based in poor functioning of the DPF cortex circuit.

Let's use a clinical example to further understand these different brain parts and how they are relevant for the psychotherapeutic process. A 52-year-old woman (let's call her Juliet) is referred for help in dealing with guilty feelings about separating from her husband. They have been married for 4 years, but she feels that her emotional needs are not being met. Recently, Juliet began an affair with a woman who demonstrates caring and affection, showers her with gifts and attention, and shares her interests. Juliet has had two previous marriages, but in all of her marriages, she was more likely to do what her husband wanted and denied her self. Her new relationship is helping her get in touch with her own needs, but she is overwhelmed by its intensity. She is also overwhelmed by a demanding professional schedule, working 70 hours per week and unable to say "no" to any work request that is made of her.

In formulating a brain-based assessment, I consider that this very intelligent woman, who appears to be grounded in her executive brain (prefrontal cortex), is really being ruled by her lower brain parts (e.g., her amygdala and nucleus accumbens; the biological domain of the transactional model). This results in an imbalance of neural circuits and an unhappy and emotionally unstable woman (the psychological domain). While we work on exploring the problematic aspects of her choice of a life partner and how this is related to her own family and parents' marriage (the social aspect), we also talk about and model things Juliet can do to structure her day and accomplish her work by delegating some tasks (the idea that she doesn't have to always be available). The latter is done to strengthen the executive functioning of her frontal cortex, which results in an enhanced sense of self-efficacy and reduced levels of stress. The reduction in overwhelming stress makes possible detailed considerations of Juliet's family history (social and spiritual aspects of the work), which included the expectation of success and stringent taboos against failure.

Juliet is encouraged to make a trip to another state, to seek out an old family home, and this also helps her to put in perspective where she has come from and where she wants to go in the future (psychologically and spiritually speaking). As she terminates treatment, Juliet reports feeling more firmly grounded (i.e., her executive functioning has been enhanced) and managing her emotions in a healthier way (i.e., lower brain parts are no longer out of control). Also, because the orbitofrontal amygdalar circuitry is better balanced, Juliet's harsh superego functioning has been modified.

Relationship and Mirror Neurons

One of the central characteristics of psychotherapy is the fact that it is conducted within the context of a therapeutic relationship. The importance of this relationship has been firmly held among practitioners, though there is little evidence to demonstrate why the relationship seems so crucial to the process. With recent new knowledge about the workings of the brain, to include a more precise biological description of the attachment relationship, it seems that we can now say that neuroscience is the missing link for understanding what makes the therapeutic relationship curative and effective.

The experience of engaging in a therapeutic relationship can alter the mind via the changes that occur in the synaptic connections among neurons (Solomon & Siegel, 2003). Viamontes and Beitman (2006) describe this relationship as being "a relationship between two brains and their bodies" (p. 214), which clearly puts the focus on what is most important. Our increasingly sophisticated understandings of the primary attachment relationship and how this colors all future relationships has led to the conclusion that the therapeutic relationship can enhance or replace an attachment relationship, based on how the right brain develops and continues to function in adulthood. The clinical relationship has always been at the core of what social workers do, and the neuroscientific revolution provides strong and scientific support for our focus on this crucial relationship. An example from practice will help to explicate.

Consider a person we will call Theresa. A 50-year-old woman, Theresa telephoned a clinical social worker and said she needed crisis counseling. She had recently lost her sister to cancer, and her aged mother was temporarily living with her, causing her much distress. Theresa and the clinician met and quickly developed an empathic relationship. The quick relationship development seemed to be based on Theresa's need for a replacement mother, because her own mother was quite aged, debilitated, and extremely invasive. Theresa and her mother were having a difficult time sharing the same living space, and there was constant shouting and bickering.

During our meetings, we talked much about Theresa's family of origin and her own yearnings for a committed relationship. I tried to focus on right brain activities (i.e., being with the client in her anger, her distress, and her mourning for a beloved sister). Direct eye contact, body movements, facial expression, and tone of voice helped me to connect with the client, as well as the mutuality of age, gender, geographical origin, and profession. I felt genuine warmth and affection for Theresa, and I believe we were able to connect "limbic brain to limbic brain" (Lewis, Amini, & Lannon, 2000). One of the interventions made was concerning the sister's will, which left her estate to my client. Theresa felt much guilt about "profiting" from her sister's death. I suggested a different choice of word, because my client changed her will several years ago and also willed her estate to her sister. This cognitive intervention seemed to be accepted by the client owing to our emotional connection and her transference to me as a "good" attachment figure. So I worked left brain to right brain, and top-down to bottom-up, to encourage neural integration.

The role of mirror neurons (noted in earlier chapters) helps explain how attunement between client and therapist gets laid down in neural structure. The topic is even being talked about in the public media. On a recent National Public Radio (NPR) program, mirror neurons were described via an example from the world of golf. The announcer noted that the mere watching of Tiger Woods' golf swing could actually improve the watcher's golf swing. This astonishing statement is said to be the result of the functioning of mirror neurons, which make possible the ability to learn complex motor skills merely by watching others perform these same skills (Hamilton, 2005). The NPR story is a simplification of what transpires in the brain, but it begins to describe what actually occurs.

Rizzolatti and Gallese (at the University of Parma, Italy) discovered these visuo-motor neurons in 1995, while studying single neurons in the brains of macaque monkeys. What they found was that a certain neuron fired when one monkey was doing something, such as reaching for a peanut. When another monkey observed the first monkey, or performed the same act, the same neuron fired in her brain as well (Music, 2005). These studies have since been translated into research on humans, where evidence of mirror neurons has been found in several brain areas, namely, Broca's area (production of speech), frontal premotor cortices, and the inferior parietal region (Cambray, 2006). What this means is that as a person observes someone else engaging in a functional behavior, certain brain areas are activated, and these are the same areas that are activated when the person performs that same behavior. The mirror neurons connect visual and motor experiences and are thought to be involved in social functions such as learning, the development of gestures and verbal language, and empathic attunement (Cozolino, 2006).

Mirror neurons are especially important for the developing infant brain, as they make possible nonverbal (implicit) learning via imitation of what is seen, heard, and felt. For example, I was meeting with a doctoral student who brought along her 4-month-old daughter. As the student and I talked, the infant awoke and started making talking-like sounds. The student had mentioned earlier that while she's working at home and talking with others on the telephone, her daughter is usually present. Perhaps this is an example of how mirror neurons had previously been activated, and they kicked in again in this instant. The infant heard and saw us talking and presumably returned to her implicit memory of mom having a conversation on the telephone, though in this case the two persons talking were in the same room. For the infant, whose mirror neurons were firing, she was learning how to be in relationship with her mother and others.

Although the mirror neuron system (MNS) was at first thought to be involved only in observing and executing an action, recently it has been found to also be involved in understanding the intentions of others (Iacoboni et al., 2005) and being able to connect emotionally with others. Cozolino (2006) says that this attunement allows us "to know others from the inside out" (p. 59). Understanding intent is linked with understanding others' emotions, which we do via our reading of social situations, including social cues. This is believed to be related to the development of language, our capacity for empathy, and the development of a theory of mind. Theory of mind can be defined as one's ability to infer the mental state of oneself and that of another person (i.e., being able to understand another's intentions; Brune, 2005). It is of interest to note that persons who have autism and schizophrenia are frequently deficient in their social awareness abilities, and theory of mind is impaired in persons who have these disorders. Recent studies of persons with autism spectrum disorder conclude that the MNS in these persons is deficient (i.e., abnormal thinning and decreased MNS activity; Dapretto et al., 2006; Hadjikhani, Joseph, Snyder, & Tager-Flusberg, 2006).

Mirror neurons make it possible for us to learn new skills by imitation; in the psychotherapeutic encounter, they make possible a genuine brain-to-brain connecting between client and clinician. Recent research suggests that there exists a possible link between the MNS and one's capacity for empathy (Gazzola, Aziz-Zadeh, & Keysers, 2006), and it provides support for the neural basis of imitation and empathy (Iacoboni, 2005; Rossi & Rossi, 2006). These studies provide much evidence for how we use these parts of our brain to connect with clients, and they with us.

How mirror neurons are involved in learning and psychotherapy is all about learning new skills, new behaviors, and new ways to modulate emotions by observing others. An example is provided by a client we will call Samson, a 48-year-old male client who has a diagnosis of schizo-affective disorder. He takes lithium carbonate and has been seen in psychotherapy for 15 years. During the first few years of treatment, Samson suffered much affective instability and was chronically suicidal, which necessitated psychiatric hospitalization at least once each year. He was living at home with his parents but wanted more independence.

The clinical social worker, in consultation with Samson and his parents, located a residential facility that seemed to fit Samson's needs. The long-range goal was for him eventually to move into his own apartment. Although his intellectual skills (left brain) had always been much in evidence, Samson's social skills and ability to modulate his feeling states (right brain) were deficient. Living in a group setting made it necessary that Samson learn how to manage relationships with others, which he did by observing his peers and how they related (activation of mirror neurons), and discussing with the clinical social worker his developing social relationships.

Over the course of several years, a strong therapeutic relationship had been established, and Samson and I used this to provide a safe and empathic environment in which he could share worries and fears that he had not been able to discuss with his overbearing and powerful father. As we talked regularly about his new-found friends, Samson began to understand the intentions of others (e.g., who could be relied on as a friend and who could not) and to develop empathy for some of his friends. This helped him to become more aware of his emotions and learn how to modulate them. He developed some real feelings for one of his less functional friends, but he also realized that the friend's unmotivated behavior angered him. It could be argued that Samson imitated my demonstrations of empathy and so was able to help his less functional friend despite his disagreement with the friend's behavior. The clinician's use of empathy was modeled for Samson via mirror neurons, which the client used to develop his own beginning empathy skills. Several years ago, Samson moved into his own apartment and has not required psychiatric hospitalization for the past 5 years.

Opportunities

The opportunities exist for social workers to develop understandings and interventions that can transform clinical social work practice. Neuroscience does promise to transform both psychotherapeutic understandings and the practice of psychotherapy. This chapter has discussed the relevance of understanding and practice to social work. It has indicated, for example, how understanding will be deepened over time as the artificial character of the distinction between mind and brain is recognized in terms of treating mental illnesses. Social work will benefit from increasing understanding of the neurobiology of psychotherapy, from deeper understanding of the relevance of neuroscience. The chapter also discussed practice relevance, talking about biological examples, recognizing neural substrates of psychotherapeutic change, and relationship and mirror neurons. There is every reason to anticipate that clinical social work, like the psychotherapies, can be enhanced to the extent that brain functioning is appreciated and absorbed into practice.

Reshaping practice is an ongoing process that involves a variety of scientific and social forces (e.g., what neuroscience makes possible and what intelligence and energy disciplines such as social work bring to a study of the new findings). It is true that the evidence from neuroscience is indeed significant and compelling. Yet developing even deeper understandings and ever more effective practice is a work in progress. Social workers should aim not only to benefit from neuroscience but also to contribute to neuroscience. It is impractical to expect that we can pull "practice rabbits" out of the hat; on the contrary, we have to invest sweat in developing the practice implications of neuro-psychotherapy. Social workers should embrace the neuroscientific opportunities realistically.

7

Linking to Social Work

Psychotropic Medications and Drugs of Abuse

Social workers and other human service professionals need to be able to provide neuro-scientifically informed interventions to assist mentally ill clients being treated with psychotropic medications. Such interventions would include some acquaintance with the recent psychopharmacology findings that relate to biological differences between different groups in terms of responding to medications; they cannot shy away from such difficult topics as the functioning of drug-metabolizing enzymes, such as the P-450 systems. They require more understanding of the possibilities of personalized and genetically informed medication and a willingness to embrace the complexities of the research (e.g., greater familiarity with placebo issues).

Mental health professionals also should be able to provide neuro-scientifically competent interventions concerning persons who take drugs of abuse such as cocaine. Such interventions should especially recognize the relevance of the brain development of children and adolescents. They require familiarity with the action of neurotransmitter systems. Acquaintance with the neurobiology of drug addiction is significant (e.g., familiarity with the effect on the frontal and prefrontal cortices and with pharmacological treatments for addiction to drugs of abuse).

The brain is central to who we are and what we do. It governs all bodily functions, and it regulates our emotions, thoughts, and behaviors. Yet competent social work practice—in relation to medications that help and drugs that hurt—should recall the transactional model. Such intervention, recognizing the significance of neuroscience, is more than a mere matter of biology.

The first part of this chapter focuses on psychotropic medications intended to help treat clients who have mental, emotional, and behavioral disorders. The second half of the chapter discusses drugs of abuse, those that hamper functioning and yet are seriously plentiful in our world. As much as possible, this chapter tries to soften the technical. But as the first section indicates, there is no denying the complexity of some pharmacological processes and of some of the descriptions. The human service professional, who is eager to be more effective in coping with medications that help and drugs that hurt, will find the challenge of understanding the complexity highly rewarding.

Psychotropic Medications That Help

The role of the social worker in working with psychiatric medications has changed significantly in the past 60-plus years. Although educating clients and families about medications and working closely with prescribing physicians continue to be important social work functions, social workers also work with clients around the meaning of medication. They also advocate for the client with other providers and larger systems, and they function as consultants, counselors, and monitors of medication (Bentley & Walsh, 2006).

To discharge this increasingly expanding role in our postgenomic era, the social worker needs the kind of neuroscientific understandings discussed in this section. The Human Genome Project, completed in 2003, "identified all of the approximately 20,000 genes in human DNA" (Bear et al., 2007, p. 32); DNA (deoxyribonucleic acid), it will be recalled, is a genetic code for the hereditary information of each individual. In our postgenomic era (after this Project), research has shifted in such directions as identifying the differential effects of medications on different groups of people. Eventually, it is anticipated that genomic research will lead to a corresponding personalized medicine. This attention to diversity has been a traditional social work value.

Let's start with social work's changing role and our ongoing attention to diversity in the postgenomic context.

Changing Social Work Roles

Since the 1950s, when chlorpromazine (thorazine) began being used in the treatment of psychoses, and soon after when the first antidepressants were introduced, social workers have been working with persons who have been prescribed psychiatric medications. In the early years, the role of the social worker with respect to medications was quite limited (i.e., serving as a resource to physicians in educating clients about their medication). In more recent years, the social work role has expanded significantly.

In recent years, clients of clinical social workers are increasingly likely to take several different medications that have been prescribed to treat several overlapping mental disorders. As a result, the psychosocial work that social workers perform has become increasingly complex, and it is generally accepted that social workers require ever greater knowledge in the area of psychopharmacology to provide effective psychosocial treatment (Farmer, Bentley, & Walsh, 2006).

Social workers have long prided themselves on having an especially strong appreciation for human diversity, and we continually strive to become knowledgeable about the unique characteristics of different ethnic, racial, gender, age, and cultural groups. As the United States' population becomes increasingly diverse, with the former majority population of Caucasians soon to become a minority group, it seems especially crucial that we enhance our understandings of the population groups that will require social work services.

Yet there is more in this postgenomic age. Biological differences are increasingly recognized as relevant to medication. For one thing, there is the matter of justice, a traditional social work concern. National Association of Social Workers' recent publications, *Institutional Racism and the Social Work Profession: A Call to Action*, and *Indicators for the Achievement of the NASW Standards for Cultural Competence*, reinforce the profession's commitment to addressing racism and social injustice through social work practice ("Diversity Documents," 2007). In the area of psychopharmacology, there is much evidence for the need to counteract institutional racism, as to how persons from different ethnic backgrounds are often misdiagnosed and/or their symptoms misunderstood by mental health clinicians of the majority culture (Adebimpe, 1981; Segal, Bola, & Watson, 1996). It is argued here that practicing social workers must be cognizant of these injustices that exist within the mental health community and be prepared to advocate for clients and families in those situations where a lack of knowledge about a person's culture and ethnicity leads to ineffective or marginalized treatment. For another thing, there is the related issue of effectiveness of individual medication. Let's turn to recent developments that highlight biological differences between ethnic groups, information that we believe social workers and other human service professionals need to know to provide up-to-date, culturally competent interventions for persons who take psychotropic medications.

Diversity in Effects

Although we have not yet reached a time of personalized medicine, social workers should recognize that there are diversities in the effects of medications between persons in different ethnic and racial groups. What is needed is an acquaintance with the pharmacodynamics and pharmacokinetics of this diversity in effects, as well as with the functioning of CYP-450 enzymes. But we should not oversimplify the effects, as if variations among the individuals within a group do not occur.

Since the 1950s, it has been known that some medications have different effects on persons based on their racial or ethnic group, but more recently, the study of individual and ethnic differences has proliferated (Relling & Hoffman, 2007). These studies have primarily been focused in four major areas: the efficacy of antipsychotic medications, of antidepressant medications, of benzodiazepines, and the adverse effects related to medications.

This brings us to the two processes that determine the effect that a medication has on the person who is taking the medication. Pharmacokinetics and pharmacodynamics are the crucial processes. Pharmacokinetics is how the body handles a drug or how it responds to the presence of the drug. Pharmacodynamics is about the effects of the drug on the body or what the drug does to the body.

Because most of the research has been conducted on pharmacokinetic processes and this determines the amount of the psychotropic medication that is available to be used by the brain, we focus on it. There are four main components of pharmacokinetics: absorption is the process by which a drug moves from the site of administration into the bloodstream; distribution is the process by which the drug travels to its desired site of action; metabolism is the process by which the body breaks down the chemical structure of the drug into derivatives that can be eliminated; and excretion is how the drug is eliminated from the body. These four pharmacokinetic processes form the basis for the development of optimal dosages and dosage regimens. Of these, metabolism is the most important, because variability in how it functions is usually what leads to interindividual and cross-ethnic variation in drug response (Lin, Smith, & Ortiz, 2001).

There are many drug-metabolizing enzymes that operate in humans, but the cytochrome P-450 system seems to be the most important for metabolism of psychotropic medications. There exist more than 20 human CYP-450 enzymes, but 4 of them are especially significant for understanding the metabolism of psychotropic medications: CYP2D6, CYP3A4, CYP1A2, and CYP2C19. These enzymes are largely influenced by genetic polymorphisms, which are fairly common mutations that change the way the enzyme functions. Different responses found among persons of certain ethnic origins who use psychotropics are supposedly the result of varying gene expression among these 4 enzymes (Lin et al., 2001; Smith, 2006). Gene expression refers to the reading of the DNA or how the genetic material gets played out (how the gene functions) based on its interactions with the environment. This process helps to determine the amount of a particular enzyme that is available to the organism. Andreasen (2001) refers to this as "gene plasticity." The implications of this plasticity are that gene expression does not remain static; rather, it is responsive to biological and nonbiological factors such as age, gender, diet, smoking, and other effects that are part of a person's culture and environment. Although researchers traditionally have looked at how genes might affect drug action, more recent studies address how medications might affect genes (Kalow, 2005).

Of the four primary enzymes that are involved in the metabolism of psychotropic medications, the CYP2D6 enzyme is one of the most important and has been extensively studied. CYP2D6 is important for the metabolism of most heterocyclic antidepressants (e.g., desipramine and nortriptyline), some of the selective serotonin reuptake inhibitors (SSRIs; e.g., paxil and prozac), and many common antipsychotics (e.g., haldol, olanzapine, risperidone). It is frequently the cause of drug-drug interactions and is highly polymorphic, meaning that it has many mutations. Seven of these are common mutations, and they comprise more than 99% of the genetic variation in this enzyme.

These mutations are especially significant, because their effects help us to classify persons in any population into four groups. The four groups are as follows: poor metabolizers are those individuals who have no 2D6 enzyme activity; intermediate metabolizers are those who have slower 2D6 enzyme activity; extensive metabolizers have enhanced enzyme activity due to no gene mutations; and ultrarapid metabolizers have duplication or multiplication of the gene, which also results in enhanced enzyme activity (Lin et al., 2001; Smith, 2006).

These categories are clinically significant. For example, a person who is a poor metabolizer or an intermediate metabolizer will no doubt have much difficulty metabolizing medications such as nortriptyline and haldol and will experience severe side effects even when given a small dose of these medications. A person who is an extensive metabolizer would have a normal response. Someone who is an ultrarapid metabolizer would be much more efficient at clearing these medications and therefore would not benefit if given a regular dose (Daly et al., 1996). Physicians and social workers who work with clients taking these medications need to keep this information in mind when deciding whether a given person is adhering to the medication as prescribed. Sometimes a history of the client's medication use can be most useful, as the taking of blood levels (even when available) can reveal nonadherence or the presence of an ultrarapid metabolizer.

These genetic variations in CYP2D6 enzyme function have been found to vary among ethnic groups. Higher rates of poor metabolizers are found among Caucasians, but this is rarely found in ethnic groups that have no European ancestry. Lower enzyme activity or intermediate metabolizers are found among persons of African and East Asian origin. Up to 70% of East Asians (i.e., Chinese, Japanese, Korean) are so categorized. Recall that an intermediate metabolizer metabolizes drugs more slowly and may have side effects at higher doses. This enzyme functioning may be related to findings that Asians require lower doses of antidepressant and antipsychotic medications for the medication to be effective and African Americans need lower doses of tricyclic antidepressants (Lin et al., 2001; Smith, 2006).

Studies have recently shown that there are fewer Mexican Americans who can be classified as poor metabolizers when compared with Caucasians. The Mexican Americans demonstrate faster rates of 2D6 activity. This is due to very low rates of gene mutations, which would result in normal metabolism and normal response to medications that are metabolized by the CYP2D6 enzymes (Mendoza et al., 2001). When the category of ultrarapid metabolizers is studied, researchers find variable rates ranging from 1% among Swedes to 5% among Spaniards. Much higher UM rates are found among Arabs and Ethiopians, in the range of 20% to 30%. This interesting difference suggests that this variant form of genetic material originated in the Middle East, spread to North Africa, and then to the Iberian peninsula (present day Spain) during the Moorish era (beginning in 711 AD). This information further suggests that approximately one fifth to one third of Ethiopians and Middle Easterners are unable to respond to regular doses of many psychotropics, but this hypothesis has not as yet been confirmed by research (Lin et al., 2001).

The other three major CYP450 enzymes that are relevant to the pharmacokinetics of psychotropic medications and are significantly influenced by genetic polymorphisms that vary across ethnic groups are CYP1A2, CYP3A4, and CYP2C19. CYP1A2 is involved in the metabolism of many medications, including luvox, haldol, olanzapine, and clozapine. Many substances can activate this enzyme. (e.g., cruciferous vegetables such as broccoli, brussels sprouts, and cabbage; char-broiled meat).

Cigarette smoking also has a large influence on the CYP1A2 enzyme, as the constituents of tobacco induce the enzyme to function in such a way that the blood concentrations of most neuroleptics and antidepressants are reduced by about 50%. As an example, a person who smokes cigarettes and also takes clozapine or haldol may find that the medication is less effective (Smith, 2006). High-protein or high-carbohydrate diets also have a significant impact on this enzyme. A high-protein diet speeds up the metabolism of certain drugs, and a high-carbohydrate diet seems to have the opposite effect. There are examples of different immigrant populations who emigrate from their home country to another, change their diets (usually to a high-protein diet) and then metabolize drugs differently (based on their new kind of dietary intake; Lin et al., 2001). This research provides some examples of how important it is to know about a person's diet and the enzymes that are involved with specific medications, when prescribing psychotropic medications. For the nonprescriber, it is also helpful to be able to educate the medication user about the effects of diet on the management of his or her medication.

The CYP3A4 enzyme is involved in the metabolism of most benzodiazepines and several of the newer antidepressants (e.g., nefazodone, mirtazapine, reboxetine) and antipsychotics (e.g., aripiprazole, quetiapine, ziprasidone). Grapefruit juice has been found to inhibit the activity of CYP3A4, which results in an increase in blood level of medications such as nefazodone and alprazolam. Gender differences have been found, and women have increased CYP3A4 activity compared to men (Brosen, 2007).

Herbal products also may modify the activity of this enzyme, as St. John's Wort was found to induce enzyme activity, thereby greatly reducing concentration of a calcium channel inhibitor (Piscitelli, Burstein, Chaitt, Alfaro, &

Falloon, 2000). Other research supports the conclusion that herbal medicines have a significant effect on the function of the drug metabolizing enzymes of the P-450 system, either by inhibiting or inducing their expression (Gurley et al., 2002). This becomes especially important when we realize that herbal medicines are used quite extensively by persons around the world and herb-drug interactions are often not considered. It is common for people to use a combination of herbal products and Western medicines, without appreciating the toxic effects that may result. Although it is assumed that herbs are natural forms of the drug-metabolizing enzymes we have been discussing and therefore would have significant interactions with other medications, the research in this area is lacking. It is hoped that in the near future, as pharmacogenetic research methodologies continue to develop, we will find much more extensive information about these interactions.

A few studies have been conducted, and their results point to some preliminary understandings. Several herbal medicines (black pepper, garlic oil, green tea, and kava) inhibit some of the P-450 enzymes, which would lead to increased blood levels of certain psychotropics, if they were taken in conjunction with the herbal products. St. John's Wort, as noted above, was found to induce enzyme activity, especially among women, which would result in reduced concentrations of the psychotropic. It was found in a recent study of older persons (ages 60 to 76) that St. John's Wort significantly induced the CYP3A4 enzyme (by 140%), garlic oil inhibited CYP2E1 activity, and ginseng inhibited CYP2D6 activity. Gurley et al. (2005) conclude that older persons also are affected by changes in CYP activity that are mediated by herbs and that the concomitant use of herbal supplements and prescription medications should be "strongly discouraged in the elderly" (p. 538).

There also is evidence of interethnic variations in the functioning of the CYP3A4 enzyme. Asian Indians, East Asians, and Mexicans have been found to have lower 3A4 activity, and African Americans and Africans are found to have higher 3A4 activity when compared with Caucasians (Smith, 2006). The CYP2C19 enzyme, which is the fourth major P-450 enzyme, is involved in the metabolism of valium and three of the SSRIs (citalopram, escitalopram, and sertraline). The most important interethnic finding seems to be that 13% to 23% of East Asians (Chinese, Japanese, Koreans) are poor metabolizers of this enzyme versus 3% to 5% of Caucasians. These differences are apparently the result of two specific mutations that were recently found on the CYP2C19 enzyme. For clinical practice, this means that persons of East Asian ancestry are particularly sensitive to medications such as diazepam, imipramine, and citalopram (Lin et al., 2001; Smith, 2006), and doses need to be monitored accordingly. The first study of Mexican Americans and CYP2C19 mutations was recently published (Luo, Poland, Lin, & Wan, 2006). The frequencies of mutations found among Mexican Americans were significantly lower than those in African Americans, Caucasians, East Asians, and Southeast Asians studied. The authors conclude that the lower number of mutations might help to explain the lower rate of poor metabolizers among Mexican Americans, as compared with the other ethnic groups.

Human service professionals should recognize, however, the falsity of the frequent assumption that all members of a specific group are the same biologically and similar psycho-socially. Some speak of Hispanics or African Americans or Asians as if they are all the same. In fact, a Hispanic may be a Guatemalan, a Honduran, a Mexican, a Peruvian, or of some other Hispanic origin. An Asian might be Korean, Chinese, or Vietnamese, all of which are unique and different cultures. Most Americans are also derived from several different ethnic groups. So it is erroneous to think that all persons who designate themselves as a particular ethnic group are the same.

There is also the fact that race and ethnicity are social constructs, with very complex meanings, and they do not measure genetic composition. By placing an individual within a specific race or ethnic category, we are hoping to place labels and characteristics on persons that help us to feel more secure (i.e., more knowledgeable). However, this kind of categorization is less helpful in describing an individual.

Let us consider a six-member American family as one example. The parents are part German, part Swiss, part Irish, and part English. The four children each identify themselves in a different way, ethnically speaking. Although all members of this family are overtly Caucasian, their ethnicity varies. The oldest child says she is German, the youngest is German-Swiss, the two middle children identify as Irish. So what is the ethnic and cultural identity of this family? It appears to be quite variable, depending on which member of the family one consults. If the members of this family completed a survey, and we tried to correlate ethnic identity with personality characteristics or other traits and attempted to correlate ethnicity with a specific environment that might influence the P-450 enzymes, we would have to conclude that there are a multiplicity of characteristics that identify this family, even though each of the children would share 50% of the same DNA.

Add to this the complexities of the meanings of race in the United States. Is anyone purely African American or American Indian or Hispanic? For a long time, we were considered to be a melting pot of different ethnicities and cultures who came to the United States; and in a sense, we have melted together, though some would argue that we have not and should not melt together. The fact is that people of different backgrounds do join together and mate, and their children are then another kind of mixture of ethnicities and races.

The significance of all of this is that each person needs to be individualized when a physician is prescribing a psychotropic medication. Although we can approach a person with some generic knowledge based on his or her ethnic identity (e.g., research reports that African Americans have a lower baseline white blood cell count than non–African Americans and therefore are not usually prescribed clozapine), we also must gather data about lifestyle, eating habits, other substances that a person uses, and beliefs and attitudes about illness and medications. Gene–environment interactions are extremely complex, and researchers have far to go in the process of finding out precisely how the genetic and the environmental interrelate.

Treatments

Human service professionals also need to be familiar with the new psychopharmacological treatments that are available for treating mental illnesses. Consider first the medications for PTSD and then treatment of depression. Note the relevance of neuroscience in understanding these processes.

In the past decade, there has been a significant increase in the number of studies conducted to determine how genetics can be used to provide more effective psychopharmacological treatments for mental illness, and also to find treatments with fewer negative side effects. Much of this basic research is being done by molecular biologists and chemists who work in the areas of cancer, heart disease, and HIV research, but these findings can then be applied to the field of psychopharmacology. This has been accompanied by the more routine collection of DNA material and its genotyping, which makes possible the study of genetic effects on drug response.

PTSD

In chapter 5, we discussed a neurodevelopmental view of trauma and PTSD and how social workers and other mental health professionals might intervene more effectively with persons experiencing this disorder. Here, the focus is on medications to treat PTSD.

Most medications that are being used are an attempt to modify the symptoms of PTSD. They include antidepressants such as monoamine oxidase inhibitors and SSRIs, especially fluoxetine and nefazodone, and antipsychotics such as risperidone as an add-on to the antidepressant. Prazosin, an alpha-1 adrenergic receptor antagonist, is also being used to effectively reduce trauma nightmares and sleep disturbances (Raskind et al., 2007). It is now understood that traumatic stress has an impact on the brain; areas involved in the stress response are the amygdala, hippocampus, and prefrontal cortex. There is increased amygdala function because the amygdala is involved in forming enhanced declarative memory for those events that are emotionally arousing. The hippocampal volume has been found to be smaller in adults with PTSD, and recently, a longitudinal study of children with a maltreatment history and PTSD symptoms also found reduced hippocampus volume (Carrion, Weems, & Reiss, 2007).

In addition to treating the debilitating symptoms of PTSD, researchers have been working for many years to find medications that will target the underlying disorder, which involves how the brain encodes new memories and keeps unwanted memories suppressed. A primary component of a traumatic event is the huge amount of stress hormones that are released (i.e., epinephrine and cortisol), and these help to solidify memories of significant events. Researchers have used rats and later humans to study the drug propranolol, to determine if it is able to alter the effect of emotional memories. Propranolol is a beta-adrenergic receptor antagonist (beta blocker) that is used primarily for the treatment of hypertension, angina, and cardiac arrhythmias. In psychiatry, beta blockers are used to treat social phobia and other anxiety disorders. To date, studies have found that propranolol impairs the consolidation (i.e., making it a fixed memory) of declarative (things we know, the "what") memory in humans (Debiec & LeDoux, 2004).

In other words, propranolol diminishes the intensity of the memory and prevents it from overwhelming the person's thoughts later. The medication supposedly works by blocking epinephrine receptors in the amygdala (Lasley, 2007). Additional studies are ongoing to determine whether propranolol can block the reconsolidation of declarative memory, as has been shown in rat studies.

If propranolol is able to block reconsolidation, this would suggest that the medication might be effective for treating intrusive memories after they have been retrieved (Debiec & LeDoux, 2004). Other studies have found that if propranolol is given to the person shortly after experiencing a trauma, it can successfully reduce symptoms of PTSD (Pitman et al., 2002; Strange, Hurlemann, & Dolan, 2003). Several studies have also found that propranolol given in rather high doses (40 mg. 3 to 4 times daily), shortly after a traumatic event (within 6 to 9 hours) effectively reduced PTSD symptoms 1 or 2 months later (Evers, 2007); these were small studies, and larger placebo-controlled studies are in process. Although much of the research on finding medications to prevent the development of PTSD and cure persons who already have the illness is extremely exciting and hopeful, it should be noted that studying how to help the brain forget is quite controversial. Some social workers object to what is called "therapeutic forgetting," because it might result in a loss of personal identity, lead to mendacity or stagnation, and because it bespeaks an intolerance toward states of distress in oneself and others. As with any medication, there are proper and improper uses, and if propranolol develops into a cure-all for PTSD, it will be tempting to use it more broadly and even to misuse it. Perhaps this is the price we must pay to help those who are suffering greatly from illnesses that might be effectively treated.

Antidepressants

Although there exist many psychotropic medications that can effectively treat depression, there remain problems with our available medications. In 2004, the Food and Drug Administration (FDA) began to require a black box warning on all antidepressants, because new evidence found a moderately increased risk for suicide and suicidal thinking in children and adolescents who used these medications. In 2006, the FDA issued a public health advisory stating that antidepressants also carry a higher risk for suicide among young adults, up to the age of 25. Older adults were exempt from this warning. Aside from the recent scare in using antidepressants with children and adolescents, psychotropic medications in general remain highly controversial for use with children and adolescents, and research using child participants has not been conducted for most of the medications being used. Because the child and adolescent brain is still forming, we do not know what biological impact the medications may have on brain formation. Another controversial issue is the psychological and social impact. Will a child or adolescent who uses psychotropics to control symptoms become accustomed to having a drug solve the problem rather than using his or her own efforts?

What makes these occurrences all the more disturbing is that suicide risk appears to be greater during the initial weeks of treatment, and most currently marketed antidepressants take 4 to 6 weeks or longer before the patient experiences any decrease in symptoms. The large-sample multicenter study sponsored by the National Institute of Mental Health, named the Sequenced Treatment Alternatives to Relieve Depression (STAR*D) reports that currently used antidepressants are only moderately effective, because remission (i.e., absence of all or most symptoms) was achieved by only 30% of people in the study. This is especially interesting, because the study included 4,000+ outpatients who are considered to be broadly representative of depressed patients in the United States (i.e., 76% Caucasians, 18% African Americans, 2% Asian, 4% other races or multiracial [13% of these were Hispanic]; Badaracco, 2007; Patoine, 2007).

Since 1988, when fluoxetine (the first SSRI) was approved, these antidepressants have become the most frequently used drugs to treat depression, and more recently, anxiety and eating disorders. In recent years, newer, atypical antidepressants have also been marketed, and these target norepinephrine and/or serotonin. But even with this large selection of antidepressants available, there remain many individuals who do not benefit from available antidepressants. It is likely that certain kinds of depression are related to genetic mutations, and until these are known for an individual, it will be impossible to prescribe a medication that fits the person's genetic makeup. Recent studies that use functional brain imaging "have identified critical neural circuits involving the amygdala and other limbic structures, prefrontal cortical regions, thalamus, and basal ganglia that modulate emotional behavior and are disturbed in primary and secondary mood disorders" (Carlson, Singh, Zarate, Drevets, & Manji, 2006, p. 25). And researchers are at work looking for new antidepressants that have a more rapid onset.

One medication being studied is ketamine, which is used in other countries as an anesthetic for children but here in the United States is primarily used on animals and by teens and young adults who snort it at raves and clubs. Ketamine is an N-methyl-d-aspartate (NMDA) receptor antagonist that is thought to target receptors of the neurotransmitter glutamate (NMDA receptors). In a study conducted at the National Institute of Mental Health Mood Disorders Research Unit, patients diagnosed with major depression were given an intravenous infusion of either ketamine hydrochloride or placebo. Results were striking: Those who received the ketamine demonstrated significant improvement in their depression symptoms within 110 minutes after injection, and results lasted for a week (Zarate et al., 2006). This is a wonderful beginning, but problems remain. Intravenous infusion is impractical for the treatment of depression, the effects appear to taper off over time, and there were some negative side effects. But researchers are very pleased to find a medication that alleviates symptoms rapidly. Zarate et al. are also studying ketamine combined with riluzole, an anticonvulsant that also acts on glutamate signaling. They are currently engaged in clinical trials to determine whether riluzole will sustain the response induced by the ketamine (Patoine, 2007). Riluzole is also being studied, in combination with lithium, as a treatment for depressed patients with bipolar disorder. Another group of researchers who were studying ketamine inadvertently came across the sedative known as scopolamine, which targets receptors for the neurotransmitter acetylcholine, and found that it also functioned as a fast-acting antidepressant. All of these results are encouraging, though new faster acting antidepressants are still a long way from routine clinical use. New treatments for bipolar disorder are also in process, because many persons with this disorder are refractory to currently available pharmacological treatments.

Complexity

Undeniably, the neuroscience of medication is complex. And undeniably, as mentioned earlier, some technical parts of this chapter are complex. But social workers and others need not shy away from the difficulties, because the benefits for improved practice are significant.

There is complexity even in the abundance of specialties and in the fascinating discoveries that have been made—and the more that are to come. Consider the complexity reflected in some specialty titles and new understandings about placebos.

Titles

Pharmacogenomics, which is a branch of pharmaceutics, is really the joining of pharmaceutics and genetics. It is the study of how the whole genome can be applied to pharmacogenetics, which focuses on the single gene, and is the study of inherited differences in drug metabolism and response. It is not surprising that the terms *pharmacogenomics* and *pharmacogenetics* are often used interchangeably, and it is difficult to precisely define either term ("Medical Encyclopedia," n.d.). Pharmacogenomics usually refers to the broad application of genomic technologies to new drug discovery and further understanding of older drugs. Pharmacogenetics is generally understood as the study of genetic variation, which results in different responses to drugs. Although pharmacogenetics looks at one or a few genes of interest, pharmacogenomics is more likely to focus on the entire genome.

Much current clinical interest is at the pharmacogenetics level, to determine how genes are involved in drug metabolism. Although the field of pharmacogenetics has existed since the 1950s, it is only recently that it has been used in clinical practice, and this is the result of findings from the Human Genome Project, which have lead to greater understanding of the genetic variability among humans. Relling and Hoffman (2007) argue that pharmacogenetics must be incorporated into the drug approval process, so that an individual's genetic makeup can be matched with the possibility of a positive or negative response to a specific drug, as opposed to the current trial-and-error method of drug choice for a specific person. This would require that DNA be collected on all participants who participate in a clinical trial to study a proposed medication, but the benefits of such research procedures seem to outweigh the greater complexity required. It is anticipated that in the future, pharmacogenomics will result in several important benefits: (a) more powerful medicines (drugs based on the proteins, enzymes, and RNA molecules that are specific to genes and diseases); (b) better, safer drugs the first time (using a patient's genetic profile to find the best available drug from the outset); (c) more accurate methods for determining appropriate dosages (rather than using weight and age to determine dosage, a person's genetic profile will determine how the medication will be processed and metabolized); (d) improvements in the development and approval of new drugs (drug trials can target specific population groups based on genetic profile); and (e) a decrease in the overall cost of health care (due to much enhanced efficacy of drug research trials and improved treatment response; Human Genome Project Information, n.d.).

Placebos

As another example of the complexity, there is some very recent research that enlarges our understanding of placebo. Much of the controlled research that is conducted uses a placebo control for clinical trials, and often, the placebo effects are equal to or greater than the substance being studied. As a result, there is great interest in finding out more about this phenomenon.

The placebo effect is understood to be a study of the psychosocial environment of the client, while also being of interest due to its biological substrates. It is increasingly of interest, because it may lead to increased self-control for individuals and because it no doubt will provide more information about how beliefs and values can shape brain processes (Benedetti, Mayberg, Wager, Stohler & Zubieta, 2005). Expectations, whether they are positive or negative, are considered to be important factors that influence behavior, and they are believed to be involved in placebo effects. How are expectations a psychological reaction, and in what ways may they also reflect a physical response?

Researchers designed a study that would focus on the nucleus accumbens, which is located in the basal ganglia part of the brain and is known to be involved in reward expectation and emotional modulation. Prior to being given a painful injection of saline solution, participants were asked how much pain relief they expected to receive from the injection. They were also told that they would be given a second injection that contained either a pain reliever or a placebo. In fact, all study participants were given a placebo injection. While the research participants were administered the painful injection of the saline solution, they underwent PET scans to measure the dopamine activity in their brain. It was found that those participants who anticipated a strong benefit in pain relief (i.e., a reward) showed increased dopamine activity immediately after being told that the pain reliever injection was imminent (Scott et al., 2007). These same participants were also more likely to report that their pain had been relieved, even though they had received a placebo injection. In the second part of this study, research participants were asked to play a gambling game that involved cash rewards. While playing the game, fMRI scans were taken to measure brain cell activity in the nucleus accumbens. Researchers found that the brain scans of those participants who expected to win demonstrated more synaptic activity in the nucleus accumbens, and these were the same participants who were placebo responders in the first part of the experiment. These findings add to the growing evidence of a physiological component to the placebo effect, which is represented by psychosocial-induced biochemical changes to the brain and body. Also of interest is how the placebo analgesic effect (i.e., placebo-induced inability to feel pain) represents an endogenous opioid network that is naturally activated (Benedetti, 2007).

Drugs That Hurt

Social workers and other human service professionals can benefit from familiarity with the neurobiology of substance abuse and addiction, interventions for drug abuse and addiction, and new drug treatment options. Knowledge of these areas will undoubtedly increase their contribution to the well-being of their clients and of society.

Although psychotropic medications are used to treat illnesses and drugs of abuse result in illnesses, in fact, we will see many of the same brain structures and neurochemical processes involved with both kinds of drugs. Even though psychotropic medications also can be abused (surveys point to increasing abuse of pain killers), we focus here on drugs that are not acquired via a physician's prescription but rather purchased on the open market (e.g., alcohol, nicotine) or purchased from illegal sources "on the street" (e.g., cocaine, marijuana, heroin, methamphetamine).

Many people, including social workers and other human service professionals, consider drug addiction and abuse to be a moral disease or a character flaw. Others refer to addiction as a disease, but this is usually defined in a vague manner and may refer to a disease of the mind or a disease of the spirit. Until recently, we have lacked clear and firm data that could help us to really understand why drug addiction might be a disease of the body. Over the past 10 years, it has been firmly established that this is a neurobiologically based illness; addiction is a chronic brain disease. Using advanced brain-imaging technology, researchers have been able to look inside the human brain and even study persons while they are ingesting a drug such as cocaine, to see what brain parts are affected and how behavior is influenced when a drug enters the brain and body. This research provides important insights into how a drug of abuse can literally capture and hold hostage various brain systems. But the effect on brain systems is just part of the explanation, and as with all brain-implicated illnesses, this also has its environmental components.

Before describing the neurobiology of drugs of abuse, we first need to recall a sense of their impact on our society. Addiction to drugs of abuse is considered to be one of our nation's biggest public health problems. Why is it such a large problem? Because the costs to our country (including lost wages, public health care costs, and costs to the criminal justice system) are $524 billion each year (Denizet-Lewis, 2006). Even if one is not a humanitarian and not interested in the shattered lives of individuals and families, this is a huge amount of money that all of us are paying for in one way or the other. A recent national survey on drug use found that 9.1% of persons age 12 or older, or an estimated 21.6 million people, are classified as being drug dependent or abusing psychoactive substances (i.e., alcohol or illicit drugs; Volkow & Li, 2005). These figures do not include compulsive gamblers, overeaters, and sex addicts, who many would also consider to be addicts. As a result, social workers are routinely encountering clients whose individual and family lives are being adversely affected by drugs of abuse.

Neurobiology of Abuse and Addiction

Because most drug experimentation and the development of addiction occurs during adolescence and in young adulthood, it is useful to begin with these developmental periods. During infancy and the first 10 years of a person's life, the frontal lobes of the brain undergo an overproduction in wiring and increase in the volume of brain tissue, which results in the formation of millions of new synapses. As puberty begins, there is a burst of neural reorganization that involves a pruning of the frontal lobes, which are the site of planning, judgment, and self-control. We also know that the prefrontal cortex is one of the last areas of the brain to mature, which doesn't occur until early adulthood (Gogtay et al., 2004). This brain structure is especially important, because it is where the cognitive or reasoning areas create connections with emotion-related areas of the brain. This is the time when we see changes in adolescents' behavior and thought processes, which frequently have an adverse effect on their ability to consistently carry through with what they had planned.

Another change that takes place in the brain during the teen years is a change in the brain's reward and pleasure centers, which results in routine, everyday activities becoming less satisfying. This helps to explain why most teenagers begin to move away from parents and family, gravitate more toward their peers, and begin to take more risks. In evolutionary terms, this is necessary for the teen to be able to find a mate who is not a close relative. However, immature judgment, negation of routine, a proclivity for risk taking, and turning toward peers may help adolescents to be more prone to addiction (Szalavitz & Volpicelli, 2005). In fact, studies have shown that persons who are not heavy users of alcohol or other drugs during their teen years and early 20s are not likely to develop an addiction later in life. To more fully address these concerns, the National Institute on Drug Abuse initiated a major research effort in 2004 to strengthen prevention and treatment of drug abuse and addiction during the critical adolescent years. A major thrust of this endeavor is to increase understanding about brain development during adolescence, how this may increase drug vulnerability, and how the use of drugs may subvert normal neurobiological maturation.

Drugs of abuse pathologically change one or more of the common neurotransmitter systems in the brain (i.e., gamma-aminobutyric acid [GABA], glutamate, acetylcholine, dopamine, serotonin, or opioid peptides). The most important of these appears to be dopamine, because drugs of abuse induce large and rapid increases in the level of dopamine in the nucleus accumbens. Dopamine is referred to as the pleasure chemical and is the primary neurotransmitter (chemical messenger) in the brain's reward system (also called the pleasure pathway or the mesolimbic dopamine pathway; see Figure 7.1). The reward system includes the ventral tegmental area, the nucleus accumbens, and the prefrontal cortex. It enables brain cells to communicate, and it affects many critical functions, including learning, memory, movement, emotional response, and feelings of pleasure and pain. Initially, the drug of abuse increases the amount of dopamine in the system, and this leads to feelings of euphoria; after regular, repeated use, the normal amount of dopamine available in the brain is reduced and the number of dopamine receptors are also diminished. As a result, the reward system is less able to respond to behaviors that would normally produce a surge of dopamine (e.g., food, sex, humor).

The result is an addicted brain in which the reward circuitry malfunctions or becomes dysregulated, and ever larger amounts of the drug are required for the person to feel a reward. Recently, researchers have also found that the initial increase in dopamine creates a craving and an expectation of a reward. Using PET scans of 18 participants who were addicted to cocaine, the level of dopamine was measured while the participants viewed two different videos, one of nature scenes and the other of people using cocaine. Dopamine levels increased while participants watched the video showing people actually using cocaine, and the level was directly related to their self-report of craving. Apparently, seeing others use cocaine makes the person think that he or she will also be rewarded with a hit of cocaine (craving has become a conditioned response). This study is especially important, as it demonstrates the connection between dopamine and cravings and provides evidence that dopamine is a basic component of addiction. Because cravings are closely related to relapse, inhibiting the increase of dopamine points to therapeutic interventions for cocaine addiction (Volkow, Wang, Telang, et al., 2006).

Other researchers also point to the dysregulation of the dopaminergic system as being crucial for the development of addiction, but new hypotheses are being studied. For example, dopamine was earlier thought to function as a signal of pleasure, but more recently, it is seen as a predictor of salience (i.e., points out what is most important and therefore what we should focus on). De-emphasizing the pleasure aspects grew out of research on nicotine, which is known to be highly addictive, causes dopamine release, but results in little euphoria (Hyman, 2005). In addition, it has been found that pleasant and unpleasant experiences can cause an increase in dopamine, and this may be due to different types of dopamine receptors (e.g., DA1 or DA2).

The amount of dopamine available in a specific area of the brain can also be related to addiction.

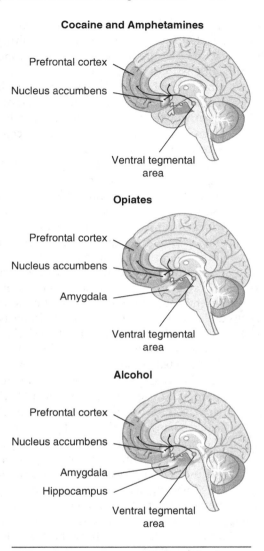

Figure 7.1   Drug Reward Systems in Brain

Studies conducted on animals and humans have found that low levels of DA2 receptors are found in those who experience drug taking as pleasurable. This might mean that fewer DA2 receptors are related to a less intense reward signal, which would lead the person to overuse the drug to feel satisfied. Knowing that low levels of DA2 might be problematic could lead to finding ways to increase DA2 receptors in humans. Volkow, Wang, Begleiter, et al. (2006) have studied families that have alcoholic and nonalcoholic members and found that the nonalcoholic members had higher-than-normal DA2 receptor availability. Alcoholism is understood as resulting from genetic and environmental factors that predispose one to vulnerability and/or protection, and this study demonstrates that DA2 receptors may protect against alcoholism. It is hypothesized that DA2 receptors, which are involved with metabolism in frontal regions of the brain, and therefore emotional reactivity and executive control, may regulate the circuits that are involved in inhibitory behavior and control of emotions. By so doing, these receptors would protect the person from becoming addicted to alcohol.

As the use of cocaine has proliferated in American society, with the resulting devastating effects on users and their families, researchers have sought better understanding of how this drug works in the body. Although dopamine continues to be important to cocaine addiction (i.e., cocaine floods the brain with dopamine), two other chemical messengers are also involved: glutamate and GABA. Glutamate is the main excitatory neurotransmitter (e.g., too much glutamate can cause a seizure), and GABA is the brain's primary inhibitory transmitter (a good analogy is a car's brakes). Glutamate is involved in memory and learning; memory and learning are also involved in addiction. Recently, it has been argued that cocaine addiction is a form of overlearning, due to too much neuroplasticity (Kalivas, 2007).

Neuroplasticity refers to the cellular changes that neurons undergo, and in cocaine addiction, this cellular learning continues to occur each time the addicted person uses cocaine. With other kinds of stimuli and rewards (e.g., food), dopamine is released initially but ceases as the person learns the appropriate response. In cocaine addiction, the user overlearns drug-seeking behavior and the thinking that is associated with drug seeking. In essence, the cellular changes continue and the brain circuits are taken over by the addiction. The brain has been flooded with dopamine, which produces a very strong memory of the intensely rewarding experience (the high) and leads to compulsive use. This process is now presumed to be involved in the neurobiological basis of drug relapse, and it is forming the basis for development of new medications to treat addiction. However, we do not currently have a good pharmacotherapy for cocaine addiction; we need to have an even better understanding about how the brain learns and how it regulates behavior (Kalivas, 2007).

Glutamate, which is neuron activating, is also thought to be important in understanding relapse (Johnson, 2004). In studies on rats, glutamate has been shown to help form trigger memories (e.g., running into a person you used to snort cocaine with), and it may help a person to access memories that prompt relapse; huge amounts of glutamate flood the system during drug-seeking behavior, and this provides nerve cell fibers with messages to activate. As such, there is believed to be an enhanced capacity for plasticity (i.e., cellular changes) in these neurons. Studies using persons who are addicted to cocaine are currently in process, and researchers are hoping to find a medication that will decrease the excess glutamate release and diminish the addicted person's compulsive drug seeking (Patoine, 2006). Alcohol also targets the glutamate system and changes the system such that withdrawal symptoms occur (shakes and anxiety) when alcohol use is stopped. These changes in the glutamate system may help the person return to alcohol use and drink even more heavily. Therefore, researchers have hypothesized that medications that would rebalance the glutamate system may help in maintaining sobriety.

Drug addiction can be defined as "compulsive drug use despite negative consequences" (Hyman, 2005, p. 1414). This is the sense in which drug dependency and addiction is so difficult to understand. When the consequences are so severe—resulting in loss of home, family, self-esteem, and even life—it is almost impossible for those who are not addicted to understand why the person persists in his or her drug use.

This is where cravings and relapse enter the picture, and much scientific endeavor has focused on understanding these two processes. In recent years, research has focused on orexin, which is a neuropeptide (i.e., a type of neurotransmitter) that is secreted by the hypothalamus (which regulates appetite and sleep/wake cycles). As an example, persons with narcolepsy have been found to be lacking in orexin. In studies on rats, orexin (also called hypocretin) has been found to be associated with addiction in rats. How it supposedly works is that stress hormones (CRF) can stimulate the production of orexin, and orexin is involved in development of drug cravings. This process is considered to be one of the ways that stress can reawaken an addiction (i.e., stress can lead to relapse). Studies show that orexin-containing neurons in the hypothalamus are necessary for the cellular changes that occur in the ventral tegmental area in the presence of cocaine. These changes include excitation of dopamine cells in the ventral tegmental area and sending of chemical signals via glutamate, which are necessary for addiction to develop. It is in this sense that orexin is referred to as "a gatekeeper of addiction" (Carr & Kalivas, 2006; Paneda, Winsky-Sommerer, Boutrel, & de Lecea, 2005).

This laboratory evidence certainly fits with what we see in practice, because relapse is one of the biggest problems for those who are drug dependent, their family, and those who work with them. These data also remind us that drug dependence and addiction is not a purely biological disease. Although there is chronic brain involvement in all addictions, there are also the psycho-social and environmental factors such as stress, which appear to provide risk or protection for drug use. Substance abuse and addiction, like other mental illnesses, can partially be understood as a misdirected attempt at self-medicating internal distress and as the result of a dysregulation of affect.

One final, important part of the neurobiology of drug addiction that needs to be discussed is the influence that drugs of abuse have on the frontal and prefrontal cortices of the brain. The latest understandings of drug addiction point to addiction as being a pathological usurpation of the processes for reward-related learning and memory. As the drug of abuse takes over (hijacks) the brain's dopamine system, cognitive processes and reasoning become impaired. The cognitive or reasoning functions of the brain are located in the frontal cortex, which also has connections with emotion-related regions of the brain (i.e., the limbic system). Specifically, these brain parts are called the *orbitofrontal cortex* and *anterior cingulate.*

The impairment in these brain parts, which is induced by the drug of abuse, leads to an overvaluing of drug reinforcers (so that alternative rewards are less powerful) and lack of inhibition for drug responses (Johnson, 2004). Using cocaine as an example, this is what occurs in the brain. Dopamine communicates with other neurons via the D1 receptors (which activate the neuron to fire) and D2 receptors (which inhibit the neuron from firing). Under normal conditions, the activating and inhibiting dopamine signals are balanced; after repeated exposure to cocaine, the balance is disrupted. The imbalance leads to an increase of inhibitory messages in the prefrontal cortex. In essence, this puts the brakes on functioning in the prefrontal cortex, which is critical for decision making. It is in this sense that the drug abusing and dependent individual loses his or her moral compass, so to speak, and is unable to behave rationally or with appropriate inhibitions, due to what is transpiring in the frontal cortex and limbic system of their brain. This diminished cognitive control results in an inability to make informed choices, as if the choice making was out of one's conscious control.

Pharmacological Treatments

There does exist a number of medications that are currently being used, with some success, for treatment of addiction, and we discuss them here. Social workers and others working with those who are addicted to drugs of abuse can benefit from knowledge of these medications and be ready for the flood of new research that is to come.

Presently, there are studies being conducted on more than 200 addiction medications. Most of these are either being conducted at the National Institute of Drug Abuse or the National Institute on Alcohol Abuse and Alcoholism or being funded by them, because the pharmaceutical industry is not very interested in developing new drugs to treat addictions, per Dr. Nora Volkow (2004), director of the National Institute on Drug Abuse. Volkow believes that we have much to learn about how drugs affect the inner workings of the brain, that this is a particularly complex endeavor, and that it includes the entire field of neuroscience research (i.e., genes, proteins, cells, brain circuits and pathways, and behavior).

Medications currently being used can be categorized as replacement therapies, dopamine transporter blockers, non-dopamine drugs, cannabinoid antagonists, corticotrophin-releasing factor antagonists, and memory blockers or enhancers (Baler & Volkow, 2006). Each of these medication subtypes is described below, with examples.

Replacement therapies, also called substitutes or agonists, bind to the same molecular targets as the drug of abuse but have different potency and pharmacokinetics. They do not provide a high as does the drug of abuse, and they prevent withdrawal symptoms and decrease opiate craving. Methadone (Dolophine), and buprenorphine (Buprenex) are examples, and they are used to treat heroin addiction. Buprenorphine (marketed as Suboxone and Subutex) was approved by the FDA in 2003 and is used to treat persons who are addicted to prescription pain medications and other opiates.

In 2000, the U.S. Congress passed the Drug Addiction Treatment Act, which allows qualified physicians to prescribe Schedule III, IV, V narcotic medications to treat opiate addiction. As a result, buprenorphine can be dispensed by physicians in private practice, thereby making it more likely to reach those who are addicted to opiates but not likely to attend a specialized drug treatment clinic. Replacement therapies that are used to treat nicotine addiction, called nicotine replacement therapy, are nicotine patches, chewing gum, and breathalyzers. Because they are medications that replace the drug of abuse and also may be addictive, these medications are controversial. But they have helped many people to lead more functional and healthier lives than if they had been using heroin or tobacco. Researchers are currently searching for an opiate agonist that can effectively treat cocaine addiction, and D1 agonists look promising.

Dopamine transporter blockers are being studied as treatments for cocaine addiction. Drugs of abuse, including cocaine, increase dopamine transmission by binding to a protein called the dopamine transporter. Blocking the effect of this transporter is seen as a potential treatment, and research on bupropion, an antidepressant that has been found effective for the treatment of nicotine addiction, is being conducted as a possible treatment for methamphetamine addiction.

Methamphetamine is a central nervous system stimulant that is extremely addictive and usually produced in clandestine laboratories across the United States. Since 1996 when the Comprehensive Methamphetamine Control Act was passed, sale of chemicals used in methamphetamine production have been controlled and many meth labs have been seized. This has resulted in the decline of U.S.-produced methamphetamine, though production in Mexico and its distribution here has increased (Office of National Drug Control Policy, n.d.). Methamphetamine has become a very popular drug among children, adolescents, and adults. The 2005 National Survey on Drug Use and Health estimates that 10.4 million Americans aged 12 or older have used methamphetamine at least once. This represents 4.3% of the U.S. population, a substantial number of people who may become addicted to this one drug.

Nondopamine drugs are currently being used in addiction treatment. The most commonly known is naltrexone, an opioid antagonist that was approved by the FDA in 1984 for treatment of opiate addiction, and in 1994 for treatment of alcoholism. Although it has been demonstrated to be effective for these two conditions and is not addicting, noncompliance is a common problem, and it is most useful for those who are highly motivated to stop using drugs (National Institute on Drug Abuse, n.d.). Since 2006, a depot form of naltrexone (Vivitrol) has been available, which can be administered as a once-monthly injection by a health care professional. This new medication is intended to be used in conjunction with psychosocial support, for those who are able to abstain from using alcohol. It is hoped that this new preparation will improve compliance.

Other nondopamine drugs that are in use and being further studied are several that involve the neurotransmitters glutamate and GABA, which are neuron activating and inhibiting, respectively. Topiramate (Topamax), classified as an anticonvulsant, has been shown to be of benefit to persons with primary alcoholism and PTSD, and for nicotine and alcohol coaddiction. It also shows promise for treatment of opiate and cocaine addictions. It blocks some effects of glutamate and potentiates the action of GABA, which fits with the theory that addictive craving is the result of too little GABA (i.e., natural brakes). It is interesting to note that at the present time, it is not clear whether less GABA is a cause of addiction or a result of drug use. A compound called N-acetylcysteine has recently been found to possibly reduce cocaine-related withdrawal symptoms and craving. This drug is an activator of cystine-glutamate exchange. Dysregulation of glutamate systems may be a factor in cocaine dependence, specifically related to euphoria, withdrawal, and craving. It can be recalled that glutamate helps to form trigger memories, and decreasing glutamatergic release may help to diminish compulsive drug seeking.

Acamprosate was approved by the FDA in 2004 and is also being used for treatment of alcohol addiction. Its action is also thought to antagonize neuronal overactivity of glutamate. In 2005, a delayed-release form of this medication, called Campral, came on the market. Acamprosate and Campral are unique in that they are the first drugs that address the underlying brain processes that occur in the disease of alcoholism. Therefore, they are quite different from naltrexone, which prevents the person from getting high and eases withdrawal but does not repair any brain damage.

Cannabinoid antagonists are being studied related to drugs of abuse, because the cannabinoid receptor system has been determined to be involved with reward, learning, and memory, all functions that are crucial to the development of drug addiction. Rimonabant blocks dopamine release in the nucleus accumbens, which is a primary reward center in the brain. Rimonabant (Acomplia) was originally developed as an antiobesity medication, whose main effect is appetite reduction. It has been approved for sale in the European Union but not yet approved by the FDA. However, Rimonabant, which is a selective type 1 cannabinoid (CB1) receptor antagonist, is being studied as a treatment for smoking cessation. Because it has demonstrated effectiveness for treatment of obesity, researchers are hopeful that it might address smokers' concerns about gaining weight if they stop smoking. In addition, brain-imaging studies have found links between addiction and obesity (Hall, 2007). In a recent review of trials conducted to determine if selective CB1 receptor antagonists would result in increased smoking cessation, the authors concluded that rimonabant appears to increase the odds for people to quit smoking (Cahill & Ussher, 2007). It has also been found to block the subjective high from marijuana and may be useful for prevention of relapse from other drugs (Volkow & Li, 2005).

Corticotropin-releasing factor antagonists are also being investigated as potential treatments for drug addiction. It is well known that stress is an important factor in many mental illnesses (e.g., the stress-vulnerability model of schizophrenia), and addiction to substances also involves the stress response. The involvement of stress in precipitating a relapse to abusing drugs, alcohol, and nicotine is especially well documented, and it is thought that a dampening of the stress response might help to prevent relapse. Specifically, withdrawal from drugs of abuse leads to the activation of brain CRF systems, and it is thought that this may result in the tremendous amounts of anxiety that are involved in drug withdrawal. Enter the CRF receptor antagonists, which have been found to block the initiation of the stress response in the brain. CRF Antalarmin is the most promising of the CRF receptor antagonists and is being studied by researchers at the National Institute on Drug Abuse.

Memory blockers or enhancers also appear to be involved in a neurobiological understanding of drug addiction, because conditioned memories have a powerful influence on the addicted person. Because of this, medications that erase or replace memories with new ones may be of use in the pharmacotherapy of drug dependence. Medications that block memory and those that enhance memory are considered in this research. For example, medications that interfere with memory formation (propranolol is an example, and also being used to treat PTSD, as discussed earlier in this chapter) might also be used to inhibit conditioned responses to cocaine. Medications that could enhance memory might be used to enhance the benefits from psychotherapeutic interventions. Memantine (Namenda) is a NDMA receptor antagonist, which is used to treat moderate to severe stages of Alzheimer's disease by blocking the effect of excess glutamate. In studies on rats, researchers have found that memantine reduced craving for alcohol, which may translate into therapeutic potential as an anticraving drug for alcohol in humans. Memantine may help to rebalance the glutamate system and be an effective treatment for alcoholism.

Other medications are also being studied in an attempt to find effective pharmacotherapeutic agents for the treatment of drug addiction. Modafinil (Provigil) is a glutamatergic agent that has been approved for the treatment of narcolepsy and is considered to be a novel stimulant that is used as an antidepressant and as a treatment for ADHD. Drugs of abuse are believed to moderate glutamate transmission in the brain, and this leads to long-lasting neuroplastic changes that may contribute to drug-seeking behavior and memories. At the present time, it remains unclear as to how glutamate transmission affects drug dependency. Does it potentiate drug-seeking behavior and drug-associated memories; or does it reduce drug reward, reinforcement, and relapse-like behavior? These questions are leading researchers toward the development of new therapeutic agents for the treatment of cocaine and amphetamine addiction, alcoholism, and weight loss (Gass & Olive, 2007).

Yet another nondopamine drug that is being studied is baclofen, which is a muscle relaxant and mimics the effects of GABA. It may help cocaine addicts to stop using, and preliminary studies show that it blocks craving in alcoholics (Baler & Volkow, 2006). Ondansetron (Zofran) is a 5-HT3 receptor antagonist, which blocks the action of serotonin. It is mainly used to treat nausea and vomiting following chemotherapy, but recent studies have shown preliminary efficacy for treatment of alcoholism. Several vaccines are also under investigation. A cocaine vaccine that slows entry of cocaine into the brain has yielded promising results, and there are three nicotine vaccines currently being developed. These vaccines work by producing antibodies to a specific drug, keeping the drug from entering the bloodstream and thereby preventing the drug of abuse from penetrating the central nervous system. The vaccines would not stop craving, so they may be of limited value, but they would make it almost impossible for an addicted person to get high from that particular drug.

Transactional Model Revisited

It is important for social workers and other mental health professionals to be aware of, at a minimum, the general features of this biological dimension, and to have some basic understanding for how brain and drug corelate. A reason is so that we may more fully use the bio-psycho-social-spiritual framework that provides the conceptual underpinning for our practice.

The brain does not operate in isolation from the rest of the person's body, and all parts are influenced by our environment. Having some understanding of the physiological impact of a drug or medication can assist us in our work with clients. But although this chapter has focused on genetic, chemical, and neurobiological processes, the psychosocial processes are of equal importance. Several physicians recently referred to pharmacotherapy as being a basically social transaction (Lin et al., 2001). This is a believable description, it seems, when we consider specific clinical examples. Haven't you encountered a person who refused to take a prescribed medication because they did not like the doctor who prescribed it? Or the person who really could not afford the medication but was too embarrassed to say so? Or the older adult whose culture considered those Westernized medicines to be pernicious? All are examples of the social interactions that take place between patient, clinician, medication, and environment. And all will determine whether or not the person uses the medication, and if so, whether or not it will be beneficial.

Consider in turn the transactional context of medications that help and of drugs that hurt.

Medications That Help

This chapter's discussion of medications that help—recent developments in pharmacogenetics—has focused almost exclusively on the biological aspects of how the body responds to the presence of a psychotropic medication when it enters the body, because pharmacokinetics is assumed to be a biological process. But we also need to talk about the other variables that are involved in this process, and these are the socio-cultural and psychological—the non-genetic factors. The role of the social worker should be as the practitioner of the transactional model.

These nonbiological factors also have a large influence on how efficiently medications are metabolized in the body and how a person responds to a medication, because the biological systems that break down the chemical structure of a medication (during the process of metabolism) are reactive to their environment. The environment, in this sense, is broad and includes many psycho-social and cultural aspects. So the factors that affect medication response include a person's age, gender, diet, intake of alcohol and/or other drugs, caffeine intake, smoking, exercise or lack thereof, disease status, use of herbal products, and personality. Other nongenetic factors that affect drug metabolism are social support, adherence to medication, and placebo effects (Lin & Smith, 2000).

It is clear that all of these factors are greatly influenced by culture and ethnicity. For instance, food intake is often culturally determined, and high or low protein, low fat, or high carbohydrate diets have an effect on the relevant enzymes that process medications. As noted earlier, we know that medicinal herbs can inhibit certain important enzymes, and members of many different cultures use herbal products in conjunction with prescribed medications. Adherence to medication is a significant problem that most clinicians and their clients have to address, and yet there is often little understanding of its causes. Bentley and Walsh (2006) review some of the vast literature on adherence and support the importance of focusing on the client's perspective (rather than the physician's), which includes the effect on one's identity of taking medication and the meaning of medication to the client.

One's beliefs and attitudes about medication are often derived from one's family of origin and one's current social contacts. We also know that in general, certain racial and ethnic groups have unique beliefs about medications. For example, Asians and Asian Americans frequently believe that it is dangerous to use Western medications on a long-term basis, and this could have a large impact on whether or not the person adheres to a medication regimen (Smith, Lin, & Mendoza, 1993). Other minority groups have had negative and racist experiences with the majority mental health system, and as a result, these persons do not trust medications or those who promote their use.

A person's response to the use of a medication is much more complex than the mere ingestion of the drug and the resultant pharmacokinetic effects.

Recall that Lin et al. (2001) noted that "pharmacotherapy is primarily and fundamentally a process of social transaction" (p. 528). This is quite a revealing statement and one that social workers need to appreciate. Are social transactions not something that we have much experience with and understanding of? Lin et al. talk about contextual factors and the interactions between patient and clinician. They admit that most physicians know much more about the biological aspects of pharmacotherapy and tend to de-emphasize the contextual. This is the place where social workers frequently enter the picture, because we work in the area of context (i.e., person in situation), and it is our task to work with clients so that they may successfully manage their use of psychotropic medications (or make an informed decision to not use medication).

One of the roles we perform in medication management is to help educate the client about their medication, why it is prescribed, and what the intended results may be. As we help the client to be a more active participant in his or her medication management and assist in his or her relationship with the prescribing physician, there is a greater likelihood that the client will adhere to the taking of medication as prescribed and that the psychosocial work we are doing with the client can also be effective.

Again, culture and ethnicity are intricately involved in this process. If the client and clinician (whether the physician or the social worker) are members of different ethnic or cultural groups, as is often the situation, there may be communication problems and misunderstandings. Perhaps the clinician has not been trained to elicit needed information in a culturally sensitive and knowledgeable way and therefore misses important data. Perhaps the client has stereotypical beliefs about medication and mental health professionals, which are grounded in his or her culture or social environment. Part of the job of the social worker, when working with clients who take medications, is to become aware of the client's beliefs about illness and medication and to assist him or her in understanding how these beliefs may influence their use of and response to medications. Sharing this information with the prescriber of medications can also lead to more effective prescribing practices, because the medication type, amount, and dosing schedule can be adjusted to best accommodate the needs of the client.

The example of psychotropic medications used to treat mental illnesses is instructive. We now know that a medication influences brain processes based on the person's genetic makeup and gene plasticity; we also know that the way a particular gene is expressed is based on biological and nonbiological factors such as age, gender, diet, smoking habits, culture, and so forth. As a result, each person who uses Luvox to treat his or her depression and anxiety will have a slightly different response and experience with this medication. This is one of the most important areas for social work input into medication use by a client. Because of the relationship we have established with our clients and our careful listening to their story, we have gathered a great deal of information that can be helpful to the prescriber of medication and the clients. Using our person-in-situation frame of reference, we are aware that gender, age, ethnicity, income, family culture, and so forth, will all affect the client's experience with medication.

The Transactional Model can help with this task, as it helps us focus on the four dimensions and how they interact with and change each other. For example, take a 40-year-old man who has a chronic schizophrenic illness and doesn't like to take his antipsychotic medication. As a social worker, we have known this client for 10 years and have talked with him often about the medication and what it means to him. He believes that the medication takes control over him and changes him as a person (psychological aspect). It also causes him to gain a large amount of weight (biological aspect). In addition, taking medication regularly stigmatizes him as a sick person (social aspect). He notes that his siblings don't take medication. The client's huge weight gain related to the antipsychotic medication influences his self-esteem (psychological domain), so we advocate with the prescribing nurse practitioner for changing the prescription to a medication with less reported weight gain. As we discuss issues of control, the client's severe paranoia comes to the fore, and we work with him to take control of his own illness management. The paranoia abates somewhat and does not disappear, but his increasing control over his own life leads to enhanced feelings of self-esteem. The new medication helps him to behave more appropriately, so a friend takes him to church with him (spiritual aspect). Attending church reinforces for him the need to take his medication as prescribed. As a result of the bio-psycho-social-spiritual domains interacting with each other and changing as a result of this interaction, this man gains some new understandings about his illness (biological, psychological, and social), the medication (biological) he uses to enhance the quality of his life, and how he can affect his own life. His life circle is now somewhat more complete.

Drugs That Hurt

Helping clients afflicted with drugs that hurt—no more than treating with medications that help—cannot be reduced to the merely biological. Treatment for drug dependency involves much more than merely finding medications that treat the symptoms of addiction or alter the brain processes that have been adversely affected by the drug of abuse.

As an example, there is the matter of the conceptualization of drug dependency and addiction. It is not a merely biological matter, and the conceptualization probably has practice implications. Drug dependency and addiction is considered by many to be a chronic brain disease, but the disease model is not accepted by everyone, and there continues to be much stigma associated with this diagnosis. First of all, drug dependency is included in the *Diagnostic and*

Statistical Manual of Mental Disorders (DSM), which from the outset puts it in a different category than diabetes or hypertension, for example. Because it is categorized in the *DSM*, it is more stigmatized than a purely medical condition, which also might be chronic. Most *DSM* diagnoses seem to place a larger dose of responsibility on the part of the patient. This is especially true for drug dependency, in which it is expected that the patient will relapse and the patient is always blamed when treatment doesn't work. Persons who are addicted receive treatment, then relapse, and then are routinely returned to the same kind of treatment, with no changes made in the therapeutic regimen, but with the hope that the treatment will succeed this time.

An example from practice will help to demonstrate the complexities involved with drug addiction and why it is helpful to approach treatment from a multidimensional perspective, such as the Transactional Model. A 21-year-old college student meets with the clinician complaining of mood instability, problems with sleeping, erratic eating behaviors, a feeling that he is unable to control his life, and history of a serious suicide attempt 5 months earlier. Almost as an aside, he mentions that he has used cocaine, heroin, hallucinogens, alcohol, and weed, but recently uses only weed and alcohol. As the family history is reviewed, we find out that his parents were divorced when he was 2 years old and that he has an older sister who lives with her mother and stepfather. His biological father is a recovering alcoholic, and though the father and son live in the same city, they rarely communicate with each other. All of his family relationships seem to be strained. The client also notes that he has been having emotional problems since the age of 10 and has been prescribed several psychotropic medications (e.g., lithium, prozac, ambien). He has many acquaintances (with whom he drinks and does drugs) but few long-term friends. He is gay but rarely dates and instead frequents bars and clubs with male and female friends.

An initial assessment would reveal that this young man is biologically vulnerable to drug dependencies, is struggling with late-adolescent identity issues, and is very unsure about moving into young adulthood (e.g., he lacks a clear sense of who he is and what he wants to do with his life). His mood instability appears to be severe enough that it affects all areas of his functioning, and it no doubt is involved in his use of substances of abuse. A plan of intervention would likely include the following: (a) referral for a medical workup to include possible need for detoxification and evaluation for psychiatric medication; (b) teaching of cognitive interventions to help the client manage his mood; (c) exploration of family issues and the possibility of reconnecting with parents as an adult; (d) education about the biology of drug use and abuse and what he can do to manage the brain changes that drugs have caused; and (e) how he can take some responsibility for how his life may unfold, even though his risk for drug dependency appears to be great. In working with this young man, the biological aspects will need to take precedence at the outset, but these will need to be coordinated with the psychological and social domains, where personality issues reside. Helping him to manage his mood symptoms and drug cravings, while trying to build and strengthen his sense of self, will be a challenge for the clinician and a long-term undertaking for the client. The relationship between the client and the clinician will need to be resilient and able to withstand the strains of addressing the biological, psychological, social, and spiritual aspects of his being.

As another example, although much research is being conducted to find new medications for the treatment of addiction, it is agreed that pharmacological and behavioral treatments that work together are required for effective treatment of drug dependence. Peter Banys (as cited in Hall, 2007) of the San Francisco Veterans Administration Medical Center thinks that addiction should be considered a heterogeneous disease with many different subtypes, each linked to a set of genes or environmental factors. For example, one's genetic vulnerability to addiction appears to be about 50% based on twin and family studies. That of course means that the remaining 50% of one's vulnerability to becoming drug dependent is based on environmental factors (i.e., being in the right place to access drugs, experiencing much stress, undergoing traumatic experiences, etc.). Banys wonders if perhaps each subtype needs a different medication or psychosocial approach.

Wow! This certainly is complex, and it reminds us that the work we do with any one person who has an addiction or dependency problem cannot be arrived at easily. The above clinical example portrays some of these challenges. Banys also suggests that the patient should not be blamed for having the disease, but he or she can be blamed for not doing something about it (Hall, 2007). This approach to addiction puts us on course to seriously consider a truly bio-psychosocial-spiritual approach to intervention. Although there are still some who are looking for the medication that will prove to be the "magic bullet" for those who are drug dependent, most researchers believe that a combined neurobiological and behavioral approach has the greatest chance of being successful (Johnson, 2004; Kalivas, 2007; Volkow & Li, 2005). One of the more unique interventions for addiction is referred to as a bio-behavioral model (Matto, 2005). This model uses dual representation theory, which is a cognitive theory used to treat PTSD (Brewin, Dagleish, & Joseph, 1996), and expressive art therapy, which adds visual processing methods to traditional CBT that is used to treat relapse prevention. Art therapy is a visual-based treatment that enables the retrieval and expression of sensory cues that are associated with addiction. This makes possible more cortical (i.e., thinking) processing to include inhibition and increased conscious control (Cozolino, 2002). The result is a combination of traditional CBT, which provides access to the brain's left hemisphere, with a creative process (guided imagery and drawing) that activates the right hemisphere. Integration of left and right hemispheres (i.e., verbal and nonverbal) has been found to be especially important in the treatment of addiction, because stress and dysregulated affect are major risk factors for relapse.

Clients' Peril

Social workers and other human service professionals neglect at their peril the insights learned from the neurobiology of medications that help and of drugs that hurt. More precisely, the peril risked is the well-being of our clients.

After all, we live in a postgenomic age. We live in the century of neuroscience.

Appendix

Teaching Suggestions

These are suggestions for incorporating book content into courses; the book will be highly suitable as a supplementary text for human behavior and clinical practice courses. This is a short starting list for neuroscience resources on the Internet and suggested discussion questions. But the list of resources is growing so exponentially that it would probably be impossible to make a comprehensive list. There is no substitute for surfing on the Web. In this, Google is very valuable.

Chapter 1

Surf

www.sfn.org This is the Web site of the Society for Neuroscience, which describes itself as the world's largest organization for understanding the brain and the nervous system. Click on "publications" (e.g., *Brain Briefings, Brain Facts)* and on "About Neuroscience" (e.g., history of neuroscience).

www.ghr.nim.nih.gov This is a guide to understanding genetic conditions. This site is a service of the U.S. National Library of Medicine.

www.genomics.energy.gov Describes the genome programs of the U.S. Department of Energy Office of Science.

www.technologyreview.com/Biotech/19328/ This site provides information about Craig Venter, who as president of Celera Genomics, competed with the Human Genome Project (U.S. Government) and sequenced the human genome using his own genetic material.

Discussion Questions

1. What is neuroscience?

2. Why is it important for social work and other human service professions?

3. What is genetics?

4. Why is genetics important for social work and other human service professions?

5. What is the neuroscientific revolution?

6. Why and how did the neuroscientific revolution occur?

Chapter 2

Surf

www.med.harvard.edu/AANLIB/home.html/ For whole brain atlas, see sites like this. Check for information on the normal brain and for images of the brain with cerebrovascular, neoplastic, degenerative, and infectious diseases.

www.images.google.com/images?hl=en&q=human+brain&um This address leads to 20 different Web sites with colorful photos of the human brain, diagrams, brain cartoons, etc.

www.brainmuseums.org For mammalian comparative brain collections, see sites like this. For example, click on "brain sections," "evolution," and "circuitry."

www.ted.com/talks/view/id/229/ This site presents Dr. Jill Bolte Taylor, a brain researcher who had a stroke 12 years ago. She describes her experience of realizing she has had a stroke.

Discussion Questions

1. What are the major components (i.e., structures) of the brain?

2. How can neurons be described, and why are they crucial to brain functioning?

3. What is distinctive about human brains?

4. What does it mean to say that "the brain is plastic?"

See Film

The video/CD PBS series on *The Secret Life of the Brain* could be shown at any time. There are five episodes: *The Baby's Brain, The Child's Brain, The Teenage Brain, The Adult Brain, and The Aging Brain.* This series would be especially useful in a human behavior course that covers the life cycle during a semester course.

Chapter 3

Surf

www.vlib.org/Biosciences Link to online resources in neurosciences; part of the WWW Virtual Library. Click on "Neurobiology."

www.bna.org.uk British Neuroscience Association. Click on, for example, "Publications." For neuroscience societies in other countries, click on "Federation of European Neuroscience Societies" at www.fens.mdc-berlin.de/

Or surf individual countries (e.g., *www.swissneuroscience.org*) The latter is a Swiss society, and click on "Newsletters."

Discussion Questions

1. What is the social domain of the transactional model?

2. What is meant by the spiritual domain?

3. How does the transactional model depict interactions between the biological, psychological, social, spiritual components, and the challenge in living?

Chapter 4

Surf

www.colchsfc.ac.uk/psychology/Copy%20of%20Links.htm For Bowlby and attachment theory.

http://video.google.com/videoplay?docid=3634664472704568591 A brief video of Mary Ainsworth on attachment and the growth of love.

http://teacher.scholastic.com/professional/bruceperry/cool.htm Titled "Keep the cool in school," this site discusses how to promote nonviolent behavior in children.

www.psychology.sunysb.edu/attachment This site reports commentary on attachment theory and research from the SUNY Stony Brook and New York Attachment Consortium. It includes attachment measures and links to attachment-related sites.

Discussion Questions

1. Is attachment theory relevant to social work practice? Why or why not?

2. How is attachment theory enriched by the findings of the neurosciences?

3. What does it mean to say that we have a social brain?

Chapter 5

Surf

www.traumaresources.org/emotional_trauma_overview.htm See this site for emotional and psychological trauma.

www.nimh.nih.gov/health/topics/post-traumatic-stress-disorder-ptsd/index.shtml For PTSD, from the National Institute of Mental Health.

www.lawandpsychiatry.com/html/hippocampus.htm For lasting effects of trauma on memory and the hippocampus.

http://www.postinstitute.com/ This is the Web site for the Post-Institute for Family-Centered Therapy, which has much information for parents and professionals.

www.ChildTrauma.org Provides descriptions of how the brain is adversely affected by experiences of trauma; offers specific suggestions for interventions that caretakers, teachers, and other human service professionals can use to calm the child.

Discussion Questions

1. How would you define trauma?

2. How is the study and treatment of trauma enriched by neuroscience?

3. Why is child neglect so detrimental to healthy development?

Chapter 6

Surf

www.neuro.psychiatryonline.org For journal and other articles on neuropsychiatry.

www.the-ins.org For the International Neuropsychological Society.

www.cogneurosociety.org For the Cognitive Neuroscience Society.

http://psychjourney.libsyn.com/indes.php?post_id=207718 This Web site offers many podcasts concerning the neuroscience of psychotherapy and an interview with Louis Cozolino.

www.neuro-psa.org.uk/npsa/index.php?module This is the Web site of the International Neuropsychoanalysis Centre, which is trying to bring together the fields of psychoanalysis, neuroscience, and psychology.

Discussion Questions

1. How do you understand the terms *mind* and *brain*?

2. How have the neurosciences affected the practice of psychotherapy?

3. What do mirror neurons have to do with the psychotherapeutic process?

4. What is your understanding of the "neurobiology of psychotherapy"?

Chapter 7

Surf

www.acnp.org For the American College of Neuropsychopharmacology.

http://www.ornl.gov/sci/techresources/Human_Genome/medicine/medicine.shtml Information about pharmacogenomics and the Human Genome.

www.nami.org/helpline/medlist.htm The National Alliance on Mental Illness provides tables of commonly prescribed medications.

www.psychservices.psychiatryonline.org Describes patterns of psychotropic medication use by race.

www.drugabuse.gov/drugpages/ This is information from the National Institute on Drug Abuse.

www.teens.drugabuse.gov/ The National Institute on Drug Abuse Web site, to educate adolescents about the science behind drug abuse.

Discussion Questions

1. Why do social workers and other nonmedical human service professionals need to know about psychotropic medications and how they work?

2. What is the importance of ethnic identity for understanding how medications work?

3. What is pharmacogenomics promising for future users of psychotropic medications?

4. How do you understand the neurobiology of addiction, and why is it important?

5. How has our knowledge of cravings and relapse been enhanced by the neurosciences?

References

Ackerman, N. (1994). *A natural history of love*. New York: Random House.

Adebimpe, V. R. (1981). Overview: White norms and psychiatric diagnosis of Black patients. *American Journal of Psychiatry, 138*, 279-285.

Adolphs, R. (2006). What is special about social cognition? In J. T. Cacioppo, P. S. Visser, & C. L. Pickett (Eds.), *Social neuroscience: People thinking about thinking people* (pp. 269-286). Cambridge, MA: MIT Press.

Ainsworth, M., Blehar, M., Waters, E., & Wall, S. (1978). *Patterns of attachment: A psychological study of the Strange Situation*. Hillsdale, NJ: Lawrence Erlbaum.

Aldwin, C. M. (1994). *Stress, coping, and development: An integrative perspective*. New York: Guilford.

Alford, J. R. (2006, September 1). *Neuroscientific advances in the study of political science*. Conference panel at the meeting of the American Political Science Association, Philadelphia.

Altman, N. (2003). Affect regulation, mentalization, and the development of the self. *Journal of Child Psychotherapy, 29*(3), 431-435.

Anda, R. F., Felitti, V. J., Bremner, J. D., Walker, J. D., Whitfield, C. H., Perry, B. D., et al. (2005, November 29). The enduring effects of abuse and related adverse experiences in childhood: A convergence of evidence from neurobiology and epidemiology. *European Archives of Psychiatry and Clinical Neuroscience*, Retrieved February 14, 2006, from http://www.springerlink.com

Anderson, R. E., & Carter, I. (1984). *Human behavior in the social environment*. New York: Aldine.

Andreasen, N. C. (2001). *Brave new brain: Conquering mental illness in the era of the genome*. New York: Oxford University Press.

Andreasen, N. C. (2005). *The creating brain: The neuroscience of genius*. New York: Dana Press.

Applegate, J. S., & Shapiro, J. R. (2005). *Neurobiology for clinical social work*. New York: W.W. Norton.

Atkins, K. (1996). Of sensory systems and the "aboutness" of mental states. *Journal of Philosophy, 93*, 337-372.

Azar, B. (2002). At the frontier of science. *Monitor on Psychology, 33*(1), 50-61.

Badaracco, M. (2007). Keeping our depressed patients in the right treatment long enough for them to get better: Some hopeful findings. *American Journal of Psychiatry, 164*(8), 1136-1139.

Bahar, A., Dudai, Y., & Ahissar, E. (2004). Neural signature of taste familiarity in the gustatory cortex of the freely behaving rat. *Journal of Neurophysiology, 92,* 3298-3308.

Baler, R. D., & Volkow, N. D. (2006). Drug addiction: The neurobiology of disrupted self-control. *Trends in Molecular Medicine, 12*(12), 559-566.

Bartels, A., & Zeki, S. (2004). The chronoarchitecture of the human brain—natural viewing conditions reveal a time-based anatomy of the brain. *Neuroimage, 22*(1), 419-433.

Bateman, A. W., & Fonagy, P. (2004). *Psychotherapy for borderline personality disorder: Mentalization based treatment.* Oxford, UK: Oxford University Press.

Baxter, L. R., Schwartz, J. M., Bergman, K. S., Szuba, M. P., Guze, B. H., Mazziotta, J. C. et al. (1992). Caudate glucose metabolic rate changes with both drug and behavior therapy for obsessive-compulsive disorder. *Archives of General Psychiatry, 49*(9), 681-689.

Bear, M. F., Connors, B. W., & Paradiso, M. A. (2007). *Neuroscience: Exploring the brain* (3rd ed.). New York: Lippincott Williams & Wilkins.

Bechara, A., & Bar-On, R. (2006). Neurological substrates of emotional and social intelligence: Evidence from patients with focal brain lesions. In J. T. Cacioppo, P. S. Visser, & C. L. Pickett (Eds.), *Social neuroscience: People thinking about thinking people* (pp. 13-40). Cambridge, MA: MIT Press.

Benedetti, F. (2007). Placebo and endogenous mechanisms of analgesia. *Handbook of Experimental Pharmacology, 177,* 393-413.

Benedetti, F., Mayberg, H. S., Wager, T. D., Stohler, C. S., & Zubieta, J. (2005). Neurobiological mechanisms of the placebo effect. *The Journal of Neuroscience, 25*(45), 10390-10402.

Bentley, K. J., & Walsh, J. (2006). *The social worker and psychotropic medication: Toward effective collaboration with mental health clients, families, and providers.* Belmont, CA: Thomson Brooks/Cole.

Berntson, G. C. (2006). Reasoning about brains. In J. T. Cacioppo, P. S. Visser, & C. L. Pickett (Eds.), *Social neuroscience: People thinking about thinking people* (pp. 1-12). Cambridge, MA: MIT Press.

Bowlby, J. (1951). *Maternal care and mental health* (World Health Organization Monograph Serial No. 2). Washington, DC: World Health Organization.

Bowlby, J. (1958). The nature of the child's tie to his mother. *International Journal of Psychoanalysis, 39,* 1-23.

Bowlby, J. (1959). Separation anxiety. *International Journal of Psychoanalysis, 41,* 1-25.

Bowlby, J. (1960). Grief and mourning in infancy and early childhood. *Psychoanalytic Study of the Child, 45,* 3-39.

Bowlby, J. (1969). *Attachment and loss: Attachment* (Vol. 1). New York: Basic Books.

Boyd, R., & Gasper, P. (1993). *The philosophy of science.* Cambridge, MA: MIT Press.

Bradley, S. J. (2000). *Affect regulation and the development of psychopathology.* New York: Guilford.

Bretherton, I. (1992). The origins of attachment theory: John Bowlby and Mary Ainsworth. *Developmental Psychology, 28*(5), 759-775.

Bretherton, I. (1999). Review of *John Bowlby: His early life. Attachment & Human Development, 1*(1), 132-136.

Brewin, C. R., Dagleish, T., & Joseph, S. (1996). A dual representation theory of posttraumatic stress disorder. *Psychological Review, 103*(4), 670-686.

British Broadcasting Corporation. (2006). *Scientists create "trust potion."* Retrieved June 30, 2006, from www.newsbbc.co.uj/2/h/health/4599299.stm

Brody, A. L., Saxena, S., Schwartz, J. M., Stoessel, P. W., Maidment, K., Phelps, M. E., et al. (1998). FDG-PET predictors of response to behavioral therapy and pharmacotherapy in obsessive compulsive disorder. *Psychiatry Research, 84*(1), 1-6.

Brody, A. L., Saxena, S., Stoessel, P., Gillies, L. A., Fairbanks, L. A., Alborzian, S., et al. (2001). Regional brain metabolic changes in patients with major depression treated with either paroxetine or interpersonal therapy. *Archives of General Psychiatry, 58*(7), 631-640.

Brooks, D. (2005, July 2). Of human bonding. *The New York Times Op-Ed,* p. 11.

Brosen, K. (2007). Sex differences in pharmacology. *Ugeskr Laeger, 169*(25), 2408-2411.

Brune, M. (2005). "Theory of mind" in schizophrenia: A review of the literature. *Schizophrenia Bulletin, 31*(1), 21-42.

Cacioppo, J. T., & Berntson, G., G. (1992). Social psychological contributions to the decade of the brain. *American Psychologist, 47*(8), 1019-1028.

Cacioppo, J. T., Visser, P. S., & Pickett, C. L. (2006). *Social neuroscience: People thinking about thinking people.* Cambridge, MA: MIT Press.

Cahill, K., & Ussher, M. (2007, July 18). Cannabinoid type 1 receptor antagonists (rimonabant) for smoking cessation. *Cochrane Database of Systematic Reviews, 4.*

Cambray, J. (2006). Towards the feeling of emergence. *Journal of Analytical Psychology, 51,* 1-20.

Carlson, P. J., Singh, J. B., Zarate, C. A., Drevets, W. C., & Manji, H. K. (2006). Neural circuitry and neuroplasticity in mood disorders: Insights for novel therapeutic targets. *NeuroRx, 3*(1), 22-41.

Carpenter, W. T. (Ed.). (2006). Proceedings, International Symposium on Schizophrenia, Bern, Switzerland, 2005 (Supplement 1). *Schizophrenia Bulletin, 32*(1), S1-S131.

Carr, D., & Kalivas, P. W. (2006). Orexin: A gatekeeper of addiction. *Nature Medicine, 12*(3), 274-276.

Carrion, V. G., Weems, C. F., & Reiss, A. L. (2007). Stress predicts brain changes in children: A pilot longitudinal study on youth stress, posttraumatic stress disorder, and the hippocampus. *Pediatrics, 119*(3), 509-516.

Carter, S. (2004). Oxytocin and the prairie vole. In J. T. Cacioppo & G. G. Berntson (Eds.), *Essays in neuroscience* (pp. 53-63). Cambridge, MA: MIT Press.

Cho, M. M., DeVries, A. C., Williams, J. R., & Carter, C. S. (1999). The effects of oxytocin and vasopressin on partner preference in male and female prairie voles. *Behavioral Neuroscience, 113*(5), 1071-1079.

Chouchourelou, A., Matsuka, T., Harber, K., & Shiffrar, M. (2006). The visual analysis of emotional reactions. *Social Neuroscience, 1*(1), 63-74.

Churchland, P. (1986). *Neurophilosophy.* Cambridge, MA: MIT Press.

Churchland, P. (2002). *Brain-wise: Studies in neurophilosophy.* Cambridge, MA: MIT Press.

Cohen, L. (2005). Neurobiology of antisociality. In C. Stough (Ed.), *Neurobiology of exceptionality* (pp. 107-124). New York: Kluwer Academic/Plenum.

Cohen, M. X., & Shaver, P. R. (2004). Avoidant attachment and hemispheric lateralization of the processing of attachment and emotion-related words. *Cognition and Emotion, 18*(6), 799-813.

Contratto, S. (2002). A feminist critique of attachment theory and evolutionary psychology. In M. Ballou & L. S. Brown (Eds.), *Rethinking mental health and disorder: Feminist perspectives* (pp. 29-47). New York: Guilford.

Cozolino, L. J. (2002). *The neuroscience of psychotherapy: Building and rebuilding the human brain*. New York: W.W. Norton.

Cozolino, L. J. (2006). *The neuroscience of human relationships: Attachment and the developing social brain*. New York: W.W. Norton.

Daly, A. K., Brockmoller, J., & Broly, F., Eichelbaum, M., Evans, W. E., Gonzalez, F. J., et al. (1996). Nomenclature for human CYP2D6 alleles. *Pharmacogenetics, 6*, 193-201.

Damasio, A. (2003). *Looking for Spinoza: Joy, sorrow, and the feeling brain*. New York: Harcourt.

Dapretto, M., Davies, M. S., Pfeifer, J. H., Scott, A. A., Sigman, M., Bookheimer, S. Y., et al. (2006). Understanding emotions in others: mirror neuron dysfunction in children with autism spectrum disorders. *Nature Neuroscience, 9*(1), 28-30.

Davidson, R. J. (1998). Anterior electrophysiological asymmetries, emotion and Depression: Conceptual and methodological conundrums. *Psychophysiology, 35,* 607-614.

Davidson, R. J. (2001). Toward a biology of personality and emotion. In A. Damasio & A. Harrington (Eds.), *Unity of knowledge: The convergence of natural and human science* (pp. 191-207). New York: New York Academy of Sciences.

Davidson, R. J. (2002). Anxiety and affective style: Role of prefrontal cortex and amygdala. *Biological Psychiatry, 51*(1), 68-80.

Davies, D. (2004). *Child development: A practitioner's guide* (2nd ed). New York: Guilford.

Dawkins, R (1976). *The selfish gene*. Oxford, UK: Oxford University Press.

De Bellis, M. D. (2005). The psychobiology of neglect. *Child Maltreatment, 10*(2), 150-172.

de Kroon, J. A. M., & Zammit, S. (2003). Neuroscience and psychodynamics. *British Journal of Psychiatry, 183*(4), 367-368.

Debiec, J., & LeDoux, J. E. (2004). Disruption of reconsolidation but not consolidation of auditory fear conditioning by noradrenergic blockade in the amygdala. *Neuroscience, 129*(2), 267-272.

Decety, J., & Keenan, J. P. (2006). *Social Neuroscience: A new journal*. Retrieved July 23, 2006, from www.social-neuroscience.com/introduction.asp

Denizet-Lewis, B. (2006, June 25). An anti-addiction pill? Message posted to RockDoc electronic mailing list, archived at http://www.RockDoc50@aol.com

Diesing, P. (1991). *How does social science work? Reflections on practice*. Pittsburgh: University of Pennsylvania Press.

Diversity Documents, Toolkit Issued. (2007, June). *NASW News, 52*(6), p. 5. Washington, DC: National Association of Social Workers.

Duncan, D. E. (2005). *The geneticist who played hoops with my DNA . . . and other masterminds from the frontiers of biotech*. New York: HarperCollins.

Eisenberg, L. (1995). The social construction of the human brain. *American Journal of Psychiatry, 152*(11), 1563-1575.

Elson, M. (1986). *Self-psychology in clinical social work*. New York: W. W. Norton & Company.

Erikson, E. H. (1950). *Childhood and society*. New York: Norton.

Etkin, A., Pittenger, C., Polan, H. J., & Kandel, E. R. (2005). Toward a neurobiology of psychotherapy: Basic science and clinical applications. *The Journal of Neuropsychiatry and Clinical Neurosciences, 17*, 145-158.

Evans, D., & Zarate, O. (1999). *Introducing evolutionary psychology*. Cambridge, UK: Icon Books.

Evers, K. (2007). Perspectives on memory manipulation: Using beta-blockers to cure post-traumatic stress disorder. *Cambridge Quarterly of Healthcare Ethics, 16*, 138-146.

Ewalt, P. (Ed.). (1980). *Toward a definition of clinical social work.* Washington, DC: National Association of Social Workers.

Eyer, D. E. (1990). Mother-infant bonding. *Human Nature: An Interdisciplinary Biosocial Perspective, 5*(1), 69-94.

Farmer, D. J. (2007). Neuro-gov: Neuroscience as catalyst. *Annals of the New York Academy of Sciences, 1118*(1), 74-89.

Farmer, R. L. (1999). Clinical HBSE concentration: A transactional model. *Journal of Social Work Education, 35*(2), 289-299.

Farmer, R. L., Bentley, K. J., & Walsh, J. (2006). Advancing social work curriculum in psychopharmacology and medication management. *Journal of Social Work Education, 42*(2), 211-229.

Farmer, R. L., & Pandurangi, A. K. (1997). Diversity in schizophrenia: Toward a richer biopsychosocial understanding for social work practice. *Health & Social Work, 22*(2), 109-116.

Feinberg, T. E., & Keenan, J. P. (2005). *The lost self: Pathologies of the brain and identity.* New York: Oxford University Press.

Fisher, H. E., Aron, A., & Mashek, D. ((2002). Defining the brain systems of lust, Romantic attraction, and attachment. *Archives of Sexual Behavior, 3*(5), 413-419.

Fonagy, P., & Bateman, A. W. (2006a). Mechanisms of change in mentalization-based treatment of BPD. *Journal of Clinical Psychology, 62*(4), 411-430.

Fonagy, P., & Bateman, A.W. (2006b). Progress in the treatment of borderline personality disorder. *The British Journal of Psychiatry, 188*, 1-3.

Forbes, H. T. (2006, July 11). But my child has been with me since birth. *Beyond Consequences eNewsletter.* Retrieved July 16, 2006, from www.beyondconsequences .com/enewsletter/issue1.html

Forbes, H. T., & Post, B. B. (2006). *Beyond consequences, logic, and control: A love based approach to helping attachment-challenged children with severe behaviors.* Orlando, FL: Beyond Consequences Institute.

Franzblau, S. H. (1999). Historicizing attachment theory: Binding the ties that bind. *Feminism and Psychology, 9*(1), 22-31.

Freud, S. (1954). *A project for a scientific psychology* (J. Strachey, Trans.). London: Imago (Original work published 1895).

Fries, A. B. W., Ziegler, T. E., Kurian, J. R., Jacoris, S., & Pollak, S. D. (2005). Early experience in humans is associated with changes in neuropeptides critical for regulating social behavior. *Proceedings of the National Academy of Sciences, 102*(47), 17237-17240.

Fujiwara, E., & Markowitsch, H. J. (2005). Autobiographical disorders. In T. E. Feinberg & J. P. Keenan (Eds.), *The lost self: Pathologies of the brain and identity* (pp. 65-80). New York: Oxford University Press.

Furmark, T., Tillfors, M., Marteinsdottir, I., Fischer, H., Pissiota, A., Langstrom, B., et al. (2002). Common changes in cerebral blood flow in patients with social phobia treated with citalopram or cognitive-behavioral therapy. *Archives of General Psychiatry, 59*(5), 425-433.

Gabbard, G. O. (2000). A neurobiologically informed perspective on psychotherapy. *British Journal of Psychiatry, 177*, 117-122.

Gabbard, G. O. (2001). Empirical evidence and psychotherapy: A growing scientific base. *American Journal of Psychiatry, 158*(1), 1-3.

Gass, J. T., & Olive, M. F. (2007, June 30). Glutamatergic substrates of drug addiction and alcoholism [Electronic version]. *Biochemical Pharmacology.* Retrieved August 25, 2007, from www.ncbi.nlm.nih.gov.proxy.library.vcu.edu/sites/entrez?Db=pubmed

Gazzola, V., Aziz-Zadeh, L., & Keysers, C. (2006). Empathy and the somatotopic auditory mirror system in humans. *Current Biology, 16*(18), 1824-1829.

Germain, C. B. (1978). General systems theory and ego psychology: An ecological perspective. *Social Science Review, 52*(4), 535-550.

Giedd, J. (2006). Inside the teenage brain. *Frontline Interview with Dr. Jay Giedd.* Retrieved August 9, 2006, from www.pbs.org/wgbh/pages/frontline/shows/teenbrain/interviews/giedd.html

Giller, E. (1999, May). *What is psychological trauma?* Workshop presented at the Annual Conference of the Maryland Mental Hygiene Administration. Retrieved May 26, 2006, from http://www.sidran.org/whatistrauma.html

Glimcher, P. W. (2003). *Decisions, uncertainty, and the brain: The science of neuro-economics.* Cambridge, MA: MIT Press.

Gogtay, N., Giedd, J. N., Lusk, L., Hayashi, K. M., Greenstein, D., Vaituzis, A. C., et al. (2004). Dynamic mapping of human cortical development during childhood through early adulthood. *Proceedings of the National Academy of Sciences, 101*(21), 8174-8179.

Goldapple, K., Segal, Z., Garson, C., Lau, M., Bieling, P., Kennedy, S., et al. (2004). Modulation of cortical-limbic pathways in major depression: Treatment-specific Effects of cognitive behavior therapy. *Archives of General Psychiatry, 61*(1), 34-41.

Goldenberg, G. (2005). Body image and the self. In T. E. Feinberg & J. P. Keenan (Eds.), *The lost self: Pathologies of the brain and identity* (pp. 81-99). New York: Oxford University Press.

Goldstein, E. G. (2007). Social work education and clinical learning: Yesterday, today, and tomorrow. *Clinical Social Work Journal, 35*(1), 15-23.

Gottesman, I. I., & Hanson, D. R. (2005). Human development: Biological and genetic processes. *Annual Review of Psychology, 56,* 263-286.

Gurley, B. J., Gardner, S. F., Hubbard, M. A., Williams, D. K., Gentry, W. B., Cui, Y., et al. (2002). Cytochrome P-450 phenotypic ratios for predicting herb-drug interactions in humans. *Clinical Pharmacology and Therapeutics, 72,* 276-287.

Gurley, B. J., Gardner, S. F., Hubbard, M. A., Williams, D. K., Gentry, W. B., Cui, Y., et al. (2005). Clinical assessment of effects of botanical supplementation on cytochrome P450 phenotypes in the elderly: St. John's wort, garlic oil, Panax ginseng and Ginkgo biloba. *Drugs Aging, 22*(6), 525-539.

Gurvits, T. V., Metzger, L. J., Lasko, N. B., Cannistraro, P. A., Tarhan, A. S., Gilbertson, M. W., et al. (2006). Subtle neurologic compromise as a vulnerability factor for combat-related posttraumatic stress disorder: Results of a twin study. *Archives of General Psychiatry, 63*(5), 571-576.

Haas, B. W., Omura, K., Amin, Z., Constable, R. T., & Canli, T. (2006). Functional connectivity with the anterior cingulateis associated with extraversion during the emotional Stroop task. *Social Neuroscience, 1*(1), 16-24.

Hadjikhani, N., Joseph, R. M., Snyder, J., & Tager-Flusberg, H. (2006). Anatomical differences in the mirror neuron system and social cognition network in autism. *Cerebral Cortex, 16*(9), 1276-1282.

Haig, D. (1993). Genetic conflicts in human pregnancy. *Quarterly Review of Biology, 68,* 495-531.

Haight, W. L., Kagle, J. D., & Black, J. E. (2003). Understanding and supporting parent child relationships during foster care visits: Attachment theory and research. *Social Work, 48*(2), 195-207.

Hall, C. T. (2007, Feb.). Riddle of addiction lures researchers. *The Dana Foundation's Brain in the News,* 5-7.

Hamilton, J. (2005, July 5). Scientists say neuron provides ability to mimic. *National Public Radio Morning Edition.* Retrieved July 5, 2005, from www.npr.org

Hamilton, W. (1964). The genetical evolution of social behavior. *Journal of Theoretical Biology, 7*(1), 1-16.

Heinzel, A., Walter, M., Schneider, F., Rotte, M., Matthiae, C. Tempelmann, C., et al. (2006). Self-related processing in the sexual domain: A parametric event-related fMRI study reveals neural activity in ventral cortical midline structures. *Social Neuroscience, 1*(1), 41-51.

Herman, J. L. (1992). *Trauma and recovery.* New York, NY: Basic Books.

Herman, J. L. (2000). *Father-daughter incest.* Cambridge, MA: Harvard University Press.

Herschkowitz, N., Kagan, J., & Zilles, K. (1997). Neurobiological bases of behavioral development in the first year. *Neuropediatrics, 28*(6), 296-306.

Hibbing, J. R., & Alford, J. R. (2006, September). *The neurological basis of representative democracy.* Paper presented at the meeting of the American Political Science Association, Philadelphia.

Hofer, M. A. (2003). The emerging neurobiology of attachment and separation: How parents shape their infant's brain and behavior. In S. W. Coates, J. L. Rosenthal, & D. S. Schechter (Eds.), *September 11: Trauma and human bonds* (pp. 191-209). Hillsdale, NJ: Analytic Press.

Human Genome Project Information. (n.d.). *Pharmacogenomics.* Retrieved July 17, 2007, from http://www.ornl.gov/sci/techresources/Human_Genome/medicine

Hyman, S. E. (2005). Addiction: A disease of learning and memory. *American Journal of Psychiatry, 162*(8), 1414-1422.

Iacoboni, M. (2005). Neural mechanisms of imitation. *Current Opinion in Neurobiology, 15*(6), 632-637.

Iacoboni, M., Molnar-Szakacs, I., Gallese, V., Buccino, G., Mazziotta, J. C., & Rizzolatti, G. (2005). Grasping the intentions of others with one's own mirror neuron system. *PLoS Biology, 3*(3), e79.

Insel, T. R. (1997). A neurobiological basis of social attachment. *American Journal of Psychiatry, 154*(6), 726-735.

Insel, T. (2006, June). *From discovery to translation: New directions in research.* Keynote address delivered at the National Alliance on Mental Illness annual convention, Washington, DC.

International Neuropsychoanalysis Society. (2008). The society: International Neuropsychoanalysis Society. Retrieved September 11, 2008, from http://www.neuropsa.org.uk/npsa/index.php?module=pagemaster&PAGE_user_op=view_page&PAGE_id=2&MMN_position=2:2

Ito, T. A., & Cacioppo, J. T. (2001). Affect and attitudes: A social neuroscience approach. In J. P. Foyas (Ed.), *Handbook of affect and social cognition* (pp. 50-74). Mahwah, NJ: Lawrence Erlbaum.

Jackson, D. C., Mueller, C. J., Dolski, I., Dalton, K. M., Nitschke, J. B., Urry, H. L., et al. (2003). Now you feel it, now you don't: Frontal brain electrical asymmetry and individual differences in emotion regulation. *Psychological Science, 14*(6), 612-617.

Johnson, H. C. (2004). *Psyche and synapse expanding worlds: The role of neurobiology in emotions, behavior, thinking, and addiction for non-scientists* (2nd ed.). Greenfield, MA: Deerfield.

Johnson, H. C., Cournoyer, D. E., Fisher, G. A., McQuillan, B. E., Moriarty, S., Richert, A. L., et al. (2000). Children's emotional and behavioral disorders: Attributions of parental responsibility by professionals. *American Journal of Orthopsychiatry, 70*(3), 327-339.

Kagan, J. (1992). Yesterday's premises, tomorrow's promises. *Developmental Psychology, 28*(6), 990-997.

Kagan, J. (1994). *Galen's prophecy: Temperament in human nature.* New York: Basic Books.

Kagan, J. (1997). Family experience and the child's development. In J. M. Notterman (Ed.), *The evolution of psychology: Fifty years of the American Psychologist* (pp. 412-421). Washington, DC: American Psychological Association.

Kagan, J., & Snidman, N. (2004). *The long shadow of temperament.* Cambridge, MA: Belknap.

Kalivas, P. W. (2007). Neurobiology of cocaine addiction: Implications for new pharmacotherapy. *The American Journal on Addictions, 16*(2), 71-78.

Kalow, W. (2005). Pharmacogenomics: Historical perspective and current status. *Methods of Molecular Biology, 311,* 3-15.

Kandel, E. R. (1979). Psychotherapy and the single synapse: The impact of psychiatric thought on neurobiological research. *New England Journal of Medicine, 301*(19), 1028-1037.

Kandel, E. R. (1998). A new intellectual framework for psychiatry. *American Journal of Psychiatry, 155,* 457-469.

Kandel, E. R. (2001). Psychotherapy and the single synapse: The impact of psychiatric thought on neurobiological research. *The Journal of Neuropsychiatry and Clinical Neurosciences, 13,* 290-300.

Konner, M. (2004). The ties that bind. *Nature, 429,* 705-707.

Krendl, A. C., Macrae, C. N., Kelley, W. M., Fugelsang, J. A., & Heatherton, T. F. (2006). The good, the bad and the ugly: An fMRI investigation of the functional anatomic correlates of stigma. *Social Neuroscience, 1*(1), 5-15.

Lasley, E. N. (2007, July/August). Memory research helps tone down what's best forgotten. *Brain Work: The Neuroscience Newsletter,* 1-3.

LeDoux, J. (1996). *The emotional brain: The mysterious underpinnings of emotional life.* New York: Simon & Schuster.

Lewis, C. S. (1960). *Four loves.* New York: Harcourt Brace.

Lewis, T., Amini, F., & Lannon, R. (2000). *A general theory of love.* New York: Random House.

Lim, M. M., Murphy, A. Z., & Young, L. J. (2004). Ventral striatopallidal oxytocin and vasopressin V1a receptors in the monogamous prairie vole. *Journal of Comparative Neurology, 468*(4), 555-570.

Lim, M. M., Wang, Z., Olazabal, D. E., Ren, X., Terwilliger, E. F., & Young, L. J. (2004). Enhanced partner preference in a promiscuous species by manipulating the expression of a single gene. *Nature, 429*(6993), 754-757.

Lin, K. M., & Smith, M. W. (2000). Psychopharmacology in the context of culture and ethnicity. *Review of Psychiatry, 19*(4), 1-36.

Lin, K. M., Smith, M. W., & Ortiz, V. (2001). Culture and psychopharmacology. *Psychiatric Clinics of North America, 24*(3), 523-538.

Linehan, M. M. (1993). *Cognitive-behavioral treatment of borderline personality disorder.* New York: Guilford.

Liu, Y., Curtis, J. T., Fowler, C. D., Spencer, C., Houpt, T., & Wang, Z. (2001). Differential expression of vasopressin, oxytocin and corticotrophin-releasing hormone messenger RNA in the paraventricular nucleus of the prairie vole brain following stress. *Journal of Neuroendicrinology, 13*(12), 1059-1065.

Luo, H. R., Poland, R. E., Lin, K. M., & Wan, Y. J. (2006). Genetic polymorphism of Cytochrome P450 2C19 in Mexican Americans: A cross-ethnic comparative study. *Clinical Pharmacology Therapeutics, 80*(1), 33-40.

Main, M. (1996). Introduction to the special section on attachment and psycho-pathology: Overview of the field of attachment. *Journal of Consulting and Clinical Psychology, 64*(2), 237-243.

Main, M., & Solomon, J. (1990). Procedures for identifying infants as disorganized/ Disoriented during the Ainsworth Strange Situation. In M. T. Greenberg, D. Cicchetti, & E. M. Cummings (Eds.), *Attachment in the preschool years* (pp. 121-160). Chicago: University of Chicago Press.

Malberg, J. E., Eisch, A. J., Nestler, E. J., & Duman, R. S. (2000). Chronic antidepressant treatment increases neurogenesis in adult rat hippocampus. *Journal of Neuroscience, 20*(24), 9104-9110.

Mascolo, M., & Fischer, K. (2004). Beyond the nature-nurture divide in development and evolution (Review of the book *Individual Development and Evolution*). *Contemporary Psychology: APA Review of Books, 48*, 842-847.

Matto, H. (2005). A bio-behavioral model of addiction treatment: Applying dual representation theory to craving management and relapse prevention. *Substance Use & Misuse, 40*(4), 529-541.

Mayberg, H. S. (2002). Modulating limbic-cortical circuits in depression: Targets of anti-depressant treatments. *Seminars in Clinical Neuropsychiatry, 7*, 255-268.

Mayberg, H. S., Brannan, S. K., Mahurin, R. K., Jerabek, P. A., Brickman, J. S., Tekell, J. L., et al. (1997). Cingulate function in depression: A potential predictor of treatment response. *Neuroreport, 8*(4), 1057-1061.

McClintock, M. K. (2004). On pheromones, vasanas, social odors and the unconscious. In J. T. Cacioppo & G. G. Berentson (Eds.), *Essays in social neuroscience* (pp. 65-76). Cambridge, MA: MIT Press.

Meaney, M. J. (2004). The nature of nurture: Maternal effects and chromatin remodeling. In J. T. Cacioppo & G. G. Berntson (Eds.), *Essays in social neuroscience* (pp. 1-14). Cambridge, MA: MIT Press.

Medical Encyclopedia: Pharmacogenetics. (n.d.). Retrieved July 17, 2007, from http://www.answers.com/topic/pharmacogenetics?cat=health

Medical Studies/Trials. (2006). *Oxytocin—don't sniff it if you want to hang on to your money.* Retrieved July 10, 2006, from www.newsmedical.net/print_article.asp?id=10597

Mega, M. S., & Cummings, J. L. (1994). Frontal-subcortical circuits and neuropsychiatric disorders. *Journal of Neuropsychiatry & Clinical Neurosciences, 6*(4), 358-370.

Mello, A. A., Mello, M. F., Carpenter, L. L., & Price, L. H. (2003). Update on stress and depression: The role of the hypothalamic-pituitary-adrenal (HPA) axis. *Review of Brasilian Psychiatry, 25*(4), 231-238.

Mendoza, R., Wan, Y. J., Poland, R. E., Smith, M., Zheng, Y., Berman, N., et al. (2001). CYP2D6 polymorphism in a Mexican American population. *Clinical Pharmacology and Therapeutics, 70*(6), 552-560.

Modell, A. H. (2003). *Imagination and the meaningful brain.* Cambridge, MA: MIT Press.

Money, J. (1986). *Lovemaps: Clinical concepts of sexual/erotic health and pathology, Paraphilia, and gender transposition of childhood, adolescence, and maturity.* New York: Irvington.

Moskowitz, M., Monk, C., Kaye, C., & Ellman, S. (Eds.). (1997). *The neurobiological and developmental basis for psychotherapeutic intervention.* Amsterdam: Jason Aronson.

Music, G. (2005). Surfacing the depths: Thoughts on imitation, resonance and growth. *Journal of Child Psychotherapy, 31*(1), 72-90.

National Institute on Drug Abuse. (n.d.). *Principles of drug addiction treatment.* Retrieved August 19, 2007, from www.drugabuse.gov/PODAT8.html

Nelson, C. A. (2000). The neurobiological bases of early intervention. In J. P. Shonkoff & S. J. Meisels (Eds.), *Handbook of early childhood intervention* (2nd ed., pp. 204-227). Cambridge, UK: Cambridge University Press.

New research shows stark differences in teen brains. (2004). *Research findings posted to IASWR listserv.* Retrieved May 11, 2004, from www.shns.com/shns/gindex2.cfm?action=detail&pk=TEENBRAINS-ABR

Oak Ridge National Laboratory. (n.d.). *Potential benefits of human genome.* Retrieved July 7, 2006, from www.ornl.gov/sci/techresources/Human_Genome/project

Ochsner, K. N., Bunge, S. A., Gross, J. J., & Gabrieli, J. D. (2002). Rethinking feelings: An FMRI study of the cognitive regulation of emotion. *Journal of Cognitive Neuroscienace, 14*(8), 1215-1229.

Ochsner, K. N., & Lieberman, M. D. (2001). The emergence of social cognitive neuroscience. *American Psychologist, 56,* 717-734.

Office of National Drug Control Policy. (n.d.). *Methamphetamine.* Retrieved August 23, 2007, from www.whitehousedrugpolicy.gov/drugfact/methamphetamine.html

Osofsky, J. D. (Ed.). (2004). *Young children and trauma.* New York: Guilford.

Palombo, J. (1985). Depletion states and self-object disorders. *Clinical Social Work Journal, 13*(1), 32-49.

Paneda, C., Winsky-Sommerer, R., Boutrel, B., & de Lecea, L. (2005). The corticotropin-releasing factor-hypocretin connection: Implications in stress response and addiction. *Drug News Pespective, 18*(4), 250-255.

Paquette, V., Levesque, J., Mensour, B., Leroux, J. M., Beaudoin, G., Bourgouin, P., et al. (2003). Change the mind and you change the brain: Effects of cognitive-behavioral therapy on the neural correlates of spider phobia. *Neuroimage, 18*(2), 401-409.

Pascal, B. (1995). *Pensees.* Section IV-277 (H. Levi, Trans.). Oxford, UK: Oxford University Press (Original work published 1670).

Patoine, B. (2006, Nov.-Dec.). Too much of a good thing: Addiction as overlearning. *BrainWork: The Neuroscience Newsletter, 16*(6), 1-3.

Patoine, B. (2007, March-April). Suicide concern highlights need for new anti-depressants. *Brain Work: The Neuroscience Newsletter,* 3-5.

Perry, B. D. (1994). Neurobiological sequelae of childhood trauma: PTSD in children. In M. Murburg (Ed.), *Catecholamine function in posttraumatic stress disorder: Emerging concepts* (pp. 233-255). Washington, DC: American Psychiatric Press.

Perry, B. D. (2002). Childhood experience and the expression of genetic potential: What childhood neglect tells us about nature and nurture. *Brain and Mind, 3,* 79-100.

Perry, B. D. (2004a). *The impact of abuse and neglect on the developing brain.* Retrieved June, 19, 2004, from http://www.teacher.scholastic.com/professional/bruceperry/abuse_neglect.htm

Perry, B. D. (2004b). Living and working with traumatized children. *The Child Trauma Academy.* Retrieved July 3, 2004, from www.ChildTrauma.org

Perry, B. D. (2004c). Neglect: How poverty of experience disrupts development. *The Child Trauma Academy.* Retrieved June 19, 2004, from www.Child Trauma.org

Perry, B. D., & Ishnella, A. (1999). Posttraumatic stress disorders in children and adolescents. *Current Opinion in Pediatrics, 11*(4), 310-322.

Perry, B. D., & Pollard, R. (1998). Homeostasis, stress, trauma, and adaptation: A neurodevelopmental view of childhood trauma. *Child and Adolescent Psychiatric Clinics of North America, 7*(1), 33-51.

Pinker, S. (1997). *How the mind works.* New York: Norton.

Piscitelli, S. C., Burstein, A. H., Chaitt, D., Alfaro, R. M., & Falloon, J. (2000). Indinavir concentrations and St. John's wort. *Lancet, 355,* 547-548.

Pitman, R. K., Sanders, K. B., Zusman, R. M., Healy, A. R., Cheema, F., Lasko, N. B., et al. (2002). Pilot study of secondary prevention of posttraumatic stress disorder with propranolol. *Biological Psychiatry, 51,* 189-192.

The Pleasure Neuron: Luxury may be habit-forming and we have the MRIs to prove it. (2005, January 30). *The New York Times Magazine,* pp. 2-3.

Project on the Decade of the Brain. (2000). *President Bush designates the 1990s as the Decade of the Brain.* Retrieved July 7, 2006, from www.loc.gov/loc/brain/

Raskind, M. A., Peskind, E. R., Hoff, D. J., Hart, K. L., Holmes, H. A., Warren, D., et al. (2007). A parallel group placebo controlled study of prazosin for trauma nightmares and sleep disturbance in combat veterans with post-traumatic stress disorder. *Biological Psychiatry, 61*(8), 928-934.

Ratna, L., & Mukergee, S. (1998). The long term effects of childhood sexual abuse: Rationale for and experience of pharmacotherapy with nefazodone. *International Journal of Psychiatric Clinic Practices, 2,* 83-95.

Reinberg, S. (2006). *HealthDay reporter.* Retrieved July 18, 2006, from www.medicinenet.com/script/main/art.asp?articlcekey=62596&pf=3&page=

Relling, M. V., & Hoffman, J. M. (2007). Should pharmacogenomic studies be required for new drug approval? *Clinical Pharmacology Therapy, 81*(3), 425-428.

Restak, R. (2003). *The new brain.* Emmaus, PA: Rodale.

Restak, R. (2006). *The naked brain: How the emerging neurosociety is changing how we live, work, and love.* New York: Harmon Books.

Reuters News Service. 2006. "Trust me" says cuddle hormone. *Australian Broadcasting Corporation.* Retrieved July 18, 2006, from www.abc.net.au/cgi-bin/common/printfriendly.pl?http://www.abc.net.au/news/newsi

Richerson, P. J., & Boyd, R. (2006). *Not by genes alone: How culture transformed human evolution.* Chicago: University of Chicago Press.

Rossi, E. L., & Rossi, K. L. (2006). The neuroscience of observing consciousness and mirror neurons in therapeutic hypnosis. *American Journal of Clinical Hypnosis, 48*(4), 263-278.

Routtenberg, A., Cantallops, I., Zaffuto, S., Serrano, P., & Namgung, U. (2000). Enhanced learning after genetic overexpression of a brain growth protein. *Proceedings of the National Academy of Sciences, 97*(13), 7657-7662.

Rubin, A., Cardenas, J., Warren, K., Pike, C., & Wambach, K. (1998). Outdated practitioner views about family culpability and severe mental disorders. *Social Work, 43,* 412-422.

Rutter, M., & English and Romanian Adoptees study team, (1998). Developmental catch-up, and deficit, following adoption after severe global early privation. *Journal of Child Psychology and Psychiatry, 39,* 465-476.

Sadock, B. J., & Sadock, V. A. (2003). *Kaplan & Sadock's synopsis of psychiatry: Behavioral sciences/clinical psychiatry* (9th ed.). Philadelphia: Lippincott Williams & Wilkins.

Saleebey, D. (1992). Biology's challenge to social work: Embodying the person-in-environment perspective. *Social Work, 37,* 112-118.

Schiemann, J. W. (2006, September 1). *Neuroscience and analytical narratives.* Paper presented at the meeting of the American Political Science Association, Philadelphia.

Schore, A. N. (1994). *Affect regulation and the origin of the self.* Hillsdale, NJ: Lawrence Erlbaum.

Schore, A. N. (2000). Attachment and the regulation of the right brain. *Attachment & Human Development, 2*(1), 23-47.

Schore, A. N. (2002). Dysregulation of the right brain: A fundamental mechanism of traumatic attachment and the psychopathogenesis of posttraumatic stress disorder. *Australian & New Zealand Journal of Psychiatry, 36*(1), 9-30.

Schore, A. N. (2003). *Affect dysregulation and disorders of the self.* New York: W. W. Norton.

Schwartz, J. M., Stoessel, P. W., Baxter, L. R., Martin, K. M., & Phelps, M. E. (1996). Systematic changes in cerebral glucose metabolic rate after successful behavior modification treatment of obsessive-compulsive disorder. *Archives of General Psychiatry, 53*(2), 109-113.

Scott, D. J., Stohler, C. S., Egnatuk, C. M., Wang, H., Koeppe, R. A., & Zubieta, J. (2007). Individual differences in reward responding explain placebo-induced expectations and effects. *Neuron, 55*(2), 325-336.

Seeman, J. (1989). Toward a model of positive health. *American Psychologist, 44*(8), 1099-1109.

Segal, S. P., Bola, J. R., & Watson, M. A. (1996). Race, quality of care, and antipsychotic prescribing practices in psychiatric emergency services. *Psychiatric Services, 47,* 282-286.

Sermabeikian, P. (1994). Our clients, ourselves: The spiritual perspective and social work practice. *Social Work, 39,* 178-183.

Shapiro, J. R., & Applegate, J. S. (2000). Cognitive neuroscience, neurobiology and affect regulation: Implications for clinical social work. *Clinical Social Work Journal, 28*(1), 9-21.

Shonkoff, J. P., & Meisels, S. J. (2000). *Handbook of early childhood intervention* (2nd ed.). New York: Cambridge University Press.

Siegel, D. J. (1999). *The developing mind: Toward a neurobiology of interpersonal experience.* New York: Guilford.

Siegel, D. J. (2001). Toward an interpersonal neurobiology of the developing mind: Attachment relationships, "mindsight," and neural integration. *Infant Mental Health Journal, 22*(1-2), 67-94.

Siegel, D. J. (2006). An interpersonal neurobiology approach to psychotherapy. *Psychiatric Annals, 36*(4), 248-256.

Smith, M. W. (2006). Ethnopsychopharmacology. In R. F. Lim (Ed.), *Clinical manual of cultural psychiatry.* Washington, DC: American Psychiatric Publishing.

Smith, M. W., Lin, K., & Mendoza, R. L. (1993). "Non-biological" issues affecting psycho-pharmacotherapy: Cultural considerations. In K. M. Lin, R. E. Poland, & G. Nakasaki (Eds.), *Psychopharmacology and psychobiology of ethnicity* (pp. 37-58). Washington, DC: American Psychiatric Press.

Society for Neuroscience. (1997). *CREB and memory* (Brain Briefing). Retrieved December 15, 2006, from www.sfn.org/index.cfm?pagename=brainBriefings_cREBAndMemory

Society for Neuroscience (1999). Insulin, the brain and memory (Brain Briefing). Retrieved December 15, 2006, from www.sfn.org/index.cfm?pagename=brain-Briefings_insulinTheBrainandMemory

Society for Neuroscience. (2000). *Bliss and the brain* (Brain Briefing). Retrieved May 28, 2007, from www.sfn.org/index.cfm?pagename=brainBriefings_blissAndtheBrain

Society for Neuroscience. (2003). *Stress and the brain* (Brain Briefing). Retrieved January 24, 2007, from www.sfn.org/index.cfm?pagename=brainBreifings_stressAnd TheBrain

Society for Neuroscience. (2004). *Memory enhancers* (Brain Briefing). Retrieved December 15, 2006, from www.sfn.org/index.cfm?pagename=brainBriefings_memoryEnhancers

Society for Neuroscience. (2006a). *Love and the brain* (Brain Briefing). Retrieved July 20, 2006, from www.sfn.org/index.cfm?pagename=brainBriefings-loveAndthebrain

Society for Neuroscience. (2006b). *Post-traumatic stress disorder: Making a difference tomorrow*. Retrieved January 24, 2007, from www.sfn.org

Solms, M. (2000). Preliminaries for an integration of psychoanalysis and neuroscience. *Annual of Psychoanalysis, 28*, 179-200.

Solomon, M., & Siegel, D. J. (Eds.). (2003). *Healing trauma: Attachment, mind, body, and brain.* New York: W.W. Norton.

Sowell, E. R., Thompson, P. M., Holmes, C. J., Jernigan, T. L., & Toga, A. W. (1999). In vivo evidence for post-adolescent brain maturation in frontal and striatal regions. *Nature Neuroscience, 2*(10), 859-861.

Sowell, E. R., Thompson, P. M., & Toga, A. W. (2004). Mapping changes through the human cortex throughout the span of life. *Neuroscientist, 10*(4), 372-392.

Spiegel, D., Bloom, J. R., Kraemer, H. C., & Gottheil, E. (1989). Effect of psychosocial treatment on survival of patients with metastatic breast cancer. *Lancet, 14*(2), 889-891.

Strange, B. A., Hurlemann, R., & Dolan, R. J. (2003). An emotion-induced retrograde amnesia in humans is amygdala-and beta-adrenergic-dependent. *Proceedings of the National Academy of Sciences, 100*, 13626-13631.

Strohman, R. C. (2003). Genetic determinism as a failing paradigm in biology and medicine: Implications for health and wellness. *Journal of Social Work Education, 39*(2), 169-191.

Stuss, D. T., Rosenblum, R. S., Malcolm, S., Christina, W., & Keenan, J. P. (2005). The frontal lobes and self-awareness. In T. E. Feinberg & J. P. Keenan (Eds.), *The lost self: Pathologies of the brain and identity* (pp. 50-64). New York: Oxford University Press.

Suomi, S. (2004). Aggression, serotonin, and gene-environment intractions in rhesus monkeys. In J. T. Cacioppo & G. G. Berentson (Eds.), *Essays in social neuroscience* (pp. 15-28). Cambridge, MA: MIT Press.

Swanson, L. W. (2003). *Brain architecture: Understanding the basic plan.* New York: Oxford University Press.

Swenson, C. R. (1995). Clinical social work. In R. L. Edwards (Ed.), *Encyclopedia of social work* (19th ed., pp. 502-512). Washington, DC: National Association of Social Workers.

Swenson, C. R., Torrey, W. C., & Koerner, K. (2002). Implementing dialectical behavior therapy. *Psychiatric Services, 53*(2), 171-178.

Szalavitz, M., & Volpicelli, J. (2005). Paradoxical profile: Alcohol's risks and benefits. *Cerebrum: The Dana Forum on Brain Science, 7*(1), 39-52.

Tancredi, L. (2005). *Hardwired behavior: What neuroscience reveals about morality.* New York: Cambridge University Press.

Taupin, P. (2005). Adult neurogenesis in the mammalian central nervous system: Functionality and potential clinical interest. *Medical Science Monitor, 11*(7), RA247-RA252.

Thomas, A., Chess, S., & Birch, H. G. (1968). *Temperament and behavior disorders in children.* New York: New York University Press.

Tizard, B., & Ree, J. (1974). A comparison of the effects of adoption, restoration to the natural mother, and continued institutionalization on the cognitive development of four-year-old children. *Child Development, 45*, 92-99.

Torrey, E. F., Bowler, A. E., Taylor, E. H., & Gottesman, I. I. (1994). *Schizophrenia and manic-depressive disorder.* New York: Basic Books.

Tronick, E. Z. (2003). Of course all relationships are unique: How co-creative processes generate unique mother-infant and patient-therapist relationships and change other relationships. *Psychoanalytic Inquiry, 23*(3), 473-491.

U.S. Department of Energy. (n.d.) *Human Genome Project information: Ethical, legal, and social issues.* Retrieved October 7, 2006, from www.ornl.gov/sci/techresources/Human_Genome/elsi/.shtml

U.S. Department of Health & Human Services, Administration for Children and Families. (2004). *Child Maltreatment 2004.* Retrieved July 10, 2006, from http://www.acf.hhs.gov/programs/cb/pubs/cm04/figures_1.htm

U.S. Senate Joint Resolution. (1990) *Joint resolution to designate the decade beginning January 1, 1990 as the "Decade of the Brain."* Retrieved July 7, 2006, from www.brainnet.org/senate.htm

Uchino, B. N., Cacioppo, J. T., Kiecolt-Glaser, J. K. (1996). The relationship between social support and physiological processes: A review with emphasis on underlying mechanisms and implications for health. *Psychological Bulletin, 119*(3), 488-531.

Urry, H. L., Nitschke, J. B., Dolski, I., Jackson, D. C., Dalton, K. M., Mueller, C. J., et al. (2004). Making a life worth living: Neural correlates of well-being. *Psychological Science, 15*(6), 367-372.

Valk, F. V., & Parisi, D. (2006, September 8). *Considerations on the neuroscience of power.* Paper presented at the meeting of the American Political Science Association, Philadelphia.

van der Kolk, B. A. (2003). The neurobiology of childhood trauma and abuse. *Child and Adolescent Psychiatric Clinics of North America, 12*, 293-317.

Van Voorhees, E., & Scarpa, A. (2004). The effects of child maltreatment on the hypothalamic-pituitary-adrenal axis. *Trauma Violence Abuse, 5*(4), 333-352.

Vaughan, C. (1997). *The talking cure.* New York: Henry Holt.

Viamontes, G. I., & Beitman, B. D. (2006). Neural substrates of psychotherapeutic change. *Psychiatric Annals, 36*(4), 238-246.

Volkow, N. D. (2004). NIDA's brain, behavior, health initiative: Multidisciplinary Exploration of the brain. *NIDA Notes, 19*(2). Retrieved July 29, 2004, from www.nida.nih.gov/NIDA_notes.html

Volkow, N. D., & Li, T. K. (2005). Drugs and alcohol: Treating and preventing abuse, addiction and their medical consequences. *Pharmacology & Therapeutics, 108*(1), 3-17.

Volkow, N. D., Wang, G. J., Begleiter, H., Porjesz, B., Fowler, J. S., Telang, F., et al. (2006). High levels of dopamine D2 receptors in unaffected members of Alcoholic families: Possible protective factors. *Archives of General Psychiatry, 63*(9), 999-1008.

Volkow, N. D., Wang, G. J., Telang, F., Fowler, J. S., Logan, J., Childress, A. R., et al. (2006, June 14). Cocaine cues and dopamine in dorsal striatum: Mechanism of craving in cocaine addiction. *Journal of Neuroscience, 26*(24), 6583-6588.

Weber, D. A., & Reynolds, C. R. (2004). Clinical perspectives on neurobiological effects of psychological trauma. *Neuropsychology Review, 14*(2), 115-129.

WebMD. (2006). *Trust potion not just fiction any more.* Retrieved July 18, 2006, from www.webmd.com/content/Article/106/108308.htm

Wexler, B. E. (2006). *Brain and culture: Neurobiology, ideology and social change.* Cambridge, MA: MIT Press.

Whitehouse, D. (2000, June 19). 'Smart gene' makes for brainy mice. *BBC News.* Retrieved July 10, 2006, from www.news.bbc.co.uk/l/hi/sci/tech/797471.stm

Wilkinson, S. R. (2003). *Coping and complaining: Attachment and the language of disease.* New York: Brunner-Routledge.

Williams, G. C. (1966). *Adaptation and natural selection.* Princeton, NJ: Princeton University Press.

Wolfe, D. L. (2003). Freud's "project" and neuroscience. *Dissertation Abstracts International, 63*(8-B), 3947.

Wylie, M. S. (2004). Mindsight: Dan Siegel offers therapists a new vision of the brain. *Psychotherapy Networker, 28*(5), 28-39.

Wylie, M. S., & Simon, R. (n.d.). *Discoveries from the black box: How the neuroscience revolution can change your practice* (Psychotherapy Networker Continuing Education Courses). Retrieved January 22, 2008, from www.psychotherapynetworker.org/index.php?category=distance_learning&sub_cat=

Young, L. J., Lim, M. M., Gingrich, B., & Insel, T. R. (2001). Cellular mechanisms of social attachment. *Hormones & Behavior, 40*(2), 133-138.

Young, L. J., & Wang, Z. (2004). The neurobiology of pair bonding. *Nature Neuroscience, 7*(10), 1048-1054.

Zarate, C. A., Singh, J. B., Carlson, P. J., Brutsche, N. E., Ameli, R., Luckenbaugh, D. A., et al. (2006). A randomized trial of an N-methyl-D-aspartate antagonist in treatment-resistant major depression. *Archives of General Psychiatry, 63*(8), 856-864.

Index

About the Author

Rosemary L. Farmer, Ph.D., LCSW, is an associate professor at the School of Social Work, Virginia Commonwealth University, where she teaches graduate courses in clinical practice, human behavior and the social environment, and psychopharmacology for social workers. She also serves as a faculty field liaison for students who are doing field work internships at various community agencies. Her MSW is from the Hunter College School of Social Work, and her Ph.D. is from the Virginia Commonwealth University School of Social Work. She has been a clinical social work practitioner for more than 30 years, with experience in state and federal psychiatric facilities, family service agencies, outpatient mental health clinics, and private practice. For example, she was a social worker at Bronx State Psychiatric Hospital; director of a psychosocial clubhouse in Montgomery County, Maryland; and a private practitioner in New York, Washington, DC, and currently in Richmond, Virginia. She has specialized in work with persons who have chronic and serious mental illnesses and their families. She has published in a variety of professional journals, on such topics as schizophrenia, gender and psychotropics, program evaluation, and the development of effective practices for social workers related to psychotropic medications. Her research interests include treating major mental illnesses and incorporating findings from the neurosciences into social work theorizing, teaching, and clinical practice.

CPSIA information can be obtained
at www.ICGtesting.com
Printed in the USA
LVHW082203250820
R16168000001B/R161680PG663657LVX4B/3

9 781412 926980